PRAISE FOR *COURAGEOUSLY EXPECTING*

"*Courageously* [. . .] elves and within their [. . .] hope and dare to believ[. . .] previous pregnancy lo[. . .]

[. . .] FOUNDER

[. . .] OF PREGNANCY AFTER LOSS SUPPORT (PALS)

"*Courageously Expecting* unfolds the emotional layers of pregnancy after loss with eloquence, grace, honesty, and sensitivity. We often hear stories about miscarriage and stillbirth, but rarely do we hear the mother's heart speaking with such raw emotion and courage. We feel seen. We feel understood. We feel a lifeline that connects us in loss and recovery. Through prompts that encourage reflection and letters to our precious babies, Albers gives us a rare opportunity to process our grief and gain the strength needed to begin once more. For every woman who has suffered a devastating pregnancy loss and for those who love these women, this illuminating read will enlighten and lift you and make you believe in the miracle of childbirth all over again."

—LISA LESHAW, MENTAL HEALTH COUNSELOR AND FREELANCE WRITER

"*Courageously Expecting* is like a comforting embrace from a friend who understands. Gently exposing the intricate aches and fears of a pregnancy after loss, Jenny Albers invites readers to step into this new season of life with expectant hearts and open hands. No matter our tomorrows, this thirty-day journey of hope and faith serves as a moving testament to the fact that joy is always on the horizon!"

—LIZ MANNEGREN, AUTHOR OF *EMBRACE: CLINGING TO CHRIST THROUGH THE PAIN OF PREGNANCY LOSS*

"This is the message we need to hear. Jenny's words are raw, beautiful, vulnerable, heartfelt, and needed. *Courageously Expecting* will bring you comfort in your pain and hope for your tomorrow. Thank you, Jenny, for sharing your story so others don't have to walk through this alone."

—LESLIE MEANS, FOUNDER OF HER VIEW FROM HOME

"Jenny Albers has crafted the most magnificent book for women who face pregnancy after loss. *Courageously Expecting* meets us at our fears and brilliantly builds our courage as we embrace the blessing within our womb. With deeply touching words she addresses every emotionally complex issue of pregnancy after loss. It's an expertly crafted book of hope, courage, and faith; a must-read for all mothers. No one should walk this journey alone. Grab Albers's hand. She is the friend you need on this walk."

—SARAH PHILPOTT, PhD, AWARD-WINNING AUTHOR OF
*LOVED BABY: 31 DEVOTIONS HELPING YOU GRIEVE AND CHERISH YOUR
CHILD AFTER PREGNANCY LOSS AND THE GROWING SEASON*

"Love, comfort, and understanding pour out of the pages of *Courageously Expecting*. In sharing her own story, Jenny helps women feel connected and understood during their own pregnancies after loss. Her words combine the hope of faith with the rawness of grief, giving her reader permission to feel both. This book is a beautiful gift to the hearts of brave mothers experiencing pregnancy after loss."

—KELSEY SCISM, A MULTIPLE-MISCARRIAGE MOM
AND WRITER AT LOVING OUR LORD

"Jenny writes with honesty and openness about one of the most vulnerable experiences a mother can have. Pregnancy after loss tests a woman's heart, her strength, and her faith—and Jenny reveals how God meets us in our heartbreak and sustains us in hope. She's the kind of friend every mom needs as she navigates the emotional journey of courageously expecting."

—CAROLYN MOORE, EDITOR-IN-CHIEF AT HER VIEW FROM HOME

"When you are pregnant after a loss, it can be difficult to hold onto hope. But with a book like Jenny Albers's *Courageously Expecting*, it's like you're holding hope in your hands. Jenny creates a safe space for you to place your fears and worries while also creating opportunities for you to channel hope into your pregnancy after loss experience. During a time that can be so lonely, this book will be your companion."

—RACHEL WHALEN, FOUNDER OF *AN UNEXPECTED FAMILY OUTING*

"In *Courageously Expecting*, Jenny Albers walks alongside the loss mom through her pregnancy after loss. She beautifully weaves her own journey with the many challenges moms face during their pregnancies after loss, giving them hope and courage to face each step. With prayers, reflections, and prompts, Jenny encourages the mom pregnant after loss to bond with her baby and cling to her faith while she waits to meet her baby. Jenny's writing wraps the pregnant after loss mom in love and validation, helping her know she is not alone."

—VALERIE R. MEEK, OPERATIONS DIRECTOR OF
PREGNANCY AFTER LOSS SUPPORT

"When you are pregnant after loss, your journey feels less like a path toward a sure destination and more like an unexpected free fall into the unknown. As a kind, empathetic companion, Jenny Albers pastors you through every step—offering you a hand to hold when the ground shakes beneath you and the free fall seems imminent. Drawing from her tender story of pregnancy after loss, Jenny uses biblical principles to remind you that hope is possible. Hope for a living baby, yes. But even more, hope in a living God. In thirty easy-to-read devotions, she candidly embraces a journey that has no guarantee. And while she doesn't know your destination, she knows the terrain. Her gentle and generous words become your lifeline, reminding you that you are anchored in more than just loss. You are anchored in truth."

—RACHEL LEWIS, AUTHOR OF *UNEXPECTING: REAL TALK ON
PREGNANCY LOSS* AND FOUNDER OF BRAVE MAMAS

COURAGEOUSLY
EXPECTING

COURAGEOUSLY EXPECTING

30 Days of Encouragement for
Pregnancy After Loss

JENNY ALBERS

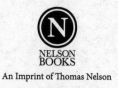

NELSON
BOOKS

An Imprint of Thomas Nelson

Courageously Expecting

© 2022 Jenny Albers

Published in Nashville, Tennessee, by Nelson Books, an imprint of Thomas Nelson. Nelson Books and Thomas Nelson are registered trademarks of HarperCollins Christian Publishing, Inc.

Thomas Nelson titles may be purchased in bulk for educational, business, fundraising, or sales promotional use. For information, please email SpecialMarkets@ThomasNelson.com.

Unless otherwise noted, Scripture quotations are taken from The Holy Bible, New International Version®, NIV®. Copyright © 1973, 1978, 1984, 2011 by Biblica, Inc.® Used by permission of Zondervan. All rights reserved worldwide. www.Zondervan.com. The "NIV" and "New International Version" are trademarks registered in the United States Patent and Trademark Office by Biblica, Inc.®

Scripture quotations marked CSB are taken from the Christian Standard Bible®. Copyright © 2017 by Holman Bible Publishers. Used by permission. Christian Standard Bible® and CSB® are federally registered trademarks of Holman Bible Publishers.

Scripture quotations marked ESV are taken from the ESV® Bible (The Holy Bible, English Standard Version®). Copyright © 2001 by Crossway, a publishing ministry of Good News Publishers. Used by permission. All rights reserved.

Scripture quotations marked MSG are taken from THE MESSAGE. Copyright © 1993, 2002, 2018 by Eugene H. Peterson. Used by permission of NavPress. All rights reserved. Represented by Tyndale House Publishers, a Division of Tyndale House Ministries.

Any internet addresses, phone numbers, or company or product information printed in this book are offered as a resource and are not intended in any way to be or to imply an endorsement by Thomas Nelson, nor does Thomas Nelson vouch for the existence, content, or services of these sites, phone numbers, companies, or products beyond the life of this book.

Library of Congress Cataloging-in-Publication Data

Names: Albers, Jenny, 1983- author.
Title: Courageously expecting : 30 days of encouragement during pregnancy after loss / Jenny Albers.
Description: Nashville, Tennessee : Nelson Books, [2022] | Summary: "Using Scripture and personal narrative, Courageously Expecting empathizes with and empowers women to face a pregnancy after loss with faith and courage, despite inevitable feelings of grief and fear that accompany life after losing a baby"-- Provided by publisher.
Identifiers: LCCN 2021019705 (print) | LCCN 2021019706 (ebook) | ISBN 9781400228232 (hardcover) | ISBN 9781400228249 (ebook)
Subjects: LCSH: Mothers--Religious life. | Pregnant women--Religious life. | Mothers--Prayers and devotions. | Pregnant women--Prayers and devotions. | Perinatal death--Religious aspects--Christianity. | Bereavement--Religious aspects--Christianity.
Classification: LCC BV4529 .A39 2022 (print) | LCC BV4529 (ebook) | DDC 248.8/66--dc23
LC record available at https://lccn.loc.gov/2021019705
LC ebook record available at https://lccn.loc.gov/2021019706

Printed in the United States of America

22 23 24 25 26 LSC 10 9 8 7 6 5 4 3 2 1

For Luke:
Thank you for loving me through the darkness
and walking in faith when I could not.
I love you.

For Annabel and Aksel:
You bring nothing but light and color to my life.
You're both my favorites.

For Micah and my baby without a name:
You've impacted my life for the better.
You are forever loved.

Contents

CONTENTS

Introduction

AN INVITATION TO CARRY
ON IN COURAGE

Motherhood was supposed to be the "happily ever after" that came second only to marriage.

When my husband and I decided we were ready to start a family, I had a vision of what that would look like—of how motherhood would go. I'd get pregnant exactly when I wanted to; we'd have three children, each three years apart; and we'd carry on unscathed, never knowing that sometimes these things don't go as planned.

My vision didn't include loss or complicated pregnancies, but those things became part of my reality anyway, and more than once the maternal happiness I'd pictured was replaced by grief.

Sure, I knew that miscarriages happen, and maybe I even had a vague understanding that sometimes babies die, though the idea of that was far too obscure for me to actually comprehend. As absurd as it sounds now, that's about all I knew. I was mostly unaware that pregnancy doesn't always go as planned. The term *stillbirth* had never been on my radar. In fact, I don't think I'd ever heard the word uttered. I'd seen something about an ectopic pregnancy in a TV drama but failed to consider that such things can happen in real life too. And as far as complications in pregnancy go, I figured morning sickness was about it.

Never could I have imagined that I would lose not one baby, but two. After a healthy and perfectly normal first pregnancy, I thought our future as a family was set, believing two more babies would join us as easily as the first one had. I had no reason to believe that the story line for my subsequent pregnancies would unfold in any way other than that of my first, ending with a baby in my arms.

But I quickly discovered that's not always the case—even when pregnancy crosses into the "safe zone" of the second trimester. Less than six weeks into my second pregnancy, a niggling pain in my lower right side vied for my attention. Though I knew better, I didn't give it much thought until it intensified to the point that I could no longer deny it—or the reality that it was likely a serious threat to my baby and my body.

After trying to push through, even running errands and engaging in my daughter's preschool dance class, I ended up writhing on the living room floor in unspeakable pain.

Something was wrong.

Hours later, in the frenzied atmosphere of the ER, I discovered I was experiencing an ectopic pregnancy. The fertilized egg, which held the very beginning stages of my baby's life, had implanted in my fallopian tube rather than my uterus, and the microscopic being inside me would never grow to see the world outside my body. With my daughter well on her way to her third birthday, the plans for my children to be spaced three years apart fell to pieces.

Nine months later, I became pregnant again. After an early ultrasound confirmed that the pregnancy was viable, and that the fertilized egg had indeed implanted where it was supposed to, I felt relieved. And yet, I still sensed that something was off. Even as my pregnancy progressed into the second trimester with no sign of trouble, I couldn't settle comfortably into the idea of bringing my baby home.

Almost one year to the date of my ectopic pregnancy, at seventeen weeks and six days pregnant, my water broke, sending my first pregnancy after loss into a tailspin of ER visits and appointments with maternal-fetal medicine specialists. For nearly three weeks, my baby and I held on. The prognosis wasn't good, and while I certainly believed that God *could* save my baby's life, I didn't get the impression that a miracle was on the horizon. In fact, I knew my baby was going to die, but I carried him until his heart and my body gave out.

Micah was born silent and still on January 31, 2015, at which point the vision I'd had for growing our family went black.

For months, my husband and I agonized over whether or not to try conceiving again. After two consecutive losses, it seemed unlikely that something would go right in a future pregnancy. Choosing to hope felt daunting, and just the *potential* of experiencing another loss felt like more than my heart could handle.

Even if I did become pregnant again, I knew that my unencumbered days of pregnancy were over. No longer did I associate carrying a child with joy and the anticipation of cradling a newborn baby against my chest. No longer would my experience of pregnancy be carefree, with the biggest concerns being how to decorate the nursery, choosing the perfect baby name, or deciding whether to buy the gray or the black car seat. No longer was success promised. No longer did becoming pregnant foretell the arrival of a new family member.

But we carried on anyway, my heart mustering the courage to hope for another living child while my head told me it was too risky. Which is why, in November 2015, when two pink lines stared at me from behind the small plastic window of a pregnancy test, I felt more bewildered than anything. I was pregnant for the fourth time. The year had started with loss and was ending with new life—but how long that life might last was a mystery.

Most people would say I was "expecting," but it was more complicated than that. What was I expecting? Was I expecting life or death? Was I expecting to leave the hospital with or without my baby? Was I expecting a full-term birth or an early death? And even in the case of a full-term birth, I knew I wasn't guaranteed to deliver a living child.

In my experience, the people familiar only with positive pregnancy outcomes were oblivious to the contradictory feelings and complexities that accompanied pregnancy after loss. It was as if becoming pregnant again erased the two previous pregnancies and the memory of the babies who once existed but didn't survive. Those around me all seemed so . . . enthusiastic. Unlike me, they automatically viewed my pregnancy as normal, as if there were nothing at all to be concerned about. To them, of course, it was a pregnancy that would end with a baby, prompting few concerns greater than sore nipples and sleepless nights.

But I knew that was only if my body cooperated.

Now, don't get me wrong. I was surrounded by people who loved me and cared about my unborn baby. But the comments meant to assure me that all would end well only made me feel misunderstood and alone.

Before loss, the idea that the emotions surrounding pregnancy could be so complicated had never entered my consciousness. Joy. Excitement. Glee. These were the feelings I was *supposed* to have. But fear, anxiety, and a sense of doom? Well, like loss, such things aren't typically discussed in the pregnancy guidebooks. But as any mom who has experienced loss knows, these feelings are the reality of pregnancy after loss, which only left me feeling more isolated in my grief.

Friend, does any of this sound familiar? The emotional turmoil, loneliness, and feeling that you don't quite fit in with other pregnant women, not to mention the grief that still lingers from losing a precious baby? Even when we cling to hope, fear is ever present and trying to pry it from our grip. But amid the swirl of our emotions is a steady God. He is our certainty when pregnancy is not.

Hope is hard. I think most women who are pregnant after loss would agree that it's the second-hardest experience of their lives. To lose a baby is the hardest, but to choose to hope for life after loss, knowing that it might not come? Well, that may as well be the definition of hard. But you know what else it is? *Courageous.* Because choosing to try again when fear is ever present and nothing is promised is not for the faint of heart.

Even when we feel misunderstood by the world at large, even when we feel alone in the uncertainty of how pregnancy will end, God sees our hardship and is right there with us. I'm not sure I've ever been as afraid or ever relied as much on God as when I was pregnant after losing Micah—when loss no longer seemed like a so-called fluke. Pages and pages of my journal, scribbled with notes about anxiety and hope and gratitude and uncertainty— along with prayers and Scripture references—are proof of my need for God. They reflect my deep fear, pronounced sorrow, breath-stopping panic, and cautious hope, with pleas to strengthen my body and my faith, laid before God in black and white.

And that's what you'll find in these pages too. The authentic and valid emotions that are part of the pregnancy-after-loss journey and the reality that God, in his goodness, has not left us to travel it alone. Because of God's presence, his grace, and his promises, we can navigate the threatening waters of pregnancy after loss with courage, despite the inevitable waves of turmoil. Because courage isn't the absence of fear; it's moving forward and tackling challenges *despite* fear.

Whether you're pregnant again or still in the stages of considering becoming so, it is my prayer that this book will remind you that you aren't alone. I'm walking with you as a mom who knows the devastation of losing a baby and the anxiety around trying to carry another one into existence.

And the God who delights in the creation of new life as much as you do walks ahead of us both.

Courageously Expecting isn't about knowing what comes next. It's about choosing to look for beauty, goodness, and hope right now, in the midst of a pregnancy so often marked by uncertainty and fear. For thirty days you'll journey with me through my own pregnancy after the loss of Micah. You'll stop to pray, reflect on how loss has colored your subsequent pregnancy, and be encouraged to move forward in faith. You'll also find letter-writing prompts to help you connect with your baby during a time in which bonding can be difficult. I don't expect that any of this will change the difficulties of your circumstances, but my hope is that it will help sustain you by showing that you are fully seen.

Friend, as you embark on this journey of pregnancy after loss, I pray you'll find the strength to carry on in courage and faith.

Day 1

THE COURAGE TO TRY AGAIN

> *For I am the LORD your God*
> *who takes hold of your right hand*
> *and says to you, Do not fear;*
> *I will help you.*
>
> —ISAIAH 41:13

The morning sun accentuated the leaves dangling outside my window, drawing my attention to stunning shades of yellow, orange, and red. The world had turned warm and golden, and though winter's bitter conditions seemed a distant memory, a chill continued to rattle my bones.

I hadn't forgotten the circumstances that had landed me in the hospital on a cold January night months earlier. In fact, the trauma and heartache of that night were still fresh as my body, heart, and mind continued to grieve the baby who was born but never took a breath. The chill of death haunted me, and the world felt cold.

The baby I had carried for over twenty weeks had slipped

silently into heaven. The delivery room was quiet—no crying, no clapping, no congratulatory shouts, no laughter—just sorrow and the hush of death. I held my baby in the palms of my hands, trying to memorize his face, his fingers and toes, his weightlessness, before returning his tiny, still body to my nurse. Luke and I named our precious, gone-too-soon baby Micah. Then we made plans for his remains and completed my discharge paperwork. I left the hospital feeling defeated, returning home with an empty womb and arms that longed to hold the child who had been formed within me. My own child had left this earth a stranger because I hadn't had the chance to meet him before his heart stopped beating.

A few weeks after that awful night, with tearful eyes and a shaking voice, I timidly asked my doctor when it would be safe to try conceiving again. She advised that I wait at least six months to allow my body, and my heart, time to recover. Thus began the months of simultaneously tracking how many weeks pregnant I *should* be while counting down the weeks to when I *could*, potentially, become pregnant again. Under normal circumstances, I would have still been counting down the weeks to my due date, to Micah's expected arrival. But Micah was already gone, and because of that there was an acute emptiness in my womb that physically hurt. Though I was eager for that emptiness to be filled, the thought of it terrified me.

The days crept by, and I watched the scenery of the natural world slowly change. Colorful tulips and sunny daffodils appeared in places that had been snow covered and barren. Carpets of lush green grass and bright dandelions were a welcome change from winter's drab landscape and spring's unpredictability, signaling the arrival of the time when, according to my doctor, it was safe to try again. The world was coming back to life all around me, and while

I longed for my womb to do the same, I wasn't yet ready to pursue another pregnancy. I knew all too well that it would never truly be safe to do so because, just like spring weather, pregnancy had proven to be anything but predictable.

After experiencing pregnancy loss, one might find it difficult to imagine that any pregnancy might have a positive outcome. Women routinely experience successful pregnancies, and babies are born alive and healthy every day, but when you're heartbroken and observing the unfolding of a story you desperately want to be a part of, those things can seem like an impossibility. When your own pregnancy has ended with the words "I'm so sorry," it becomes all too easy to believe that a normal pregnancy is impossible—at least for you.

The aftermath of loss continued to contaminate my life, even when the window to try again finally opened, allowing the air of possibility to drift in. I continued to see pregnancy through the shadow of loss. I knew how fragile the experience could be and how easily it could break my heart—again. I was afraid to take another chance on a pregnancy that wouldn't be guaranteed, but by the time autumn's splendor arrived—three months after I'd been given the go-ahead to try again—I knew I was as ready as I would ever be. The trees displayed their most brilliant colors, yet the beauty was veiled by my fear. I was afraid another pregnancy would leave me shrouded in a thicker, more suffocating veil of darkness. If things had gone as planned, I would have been holding a baby in my arms as the leaves crisped and the air cooled. Just as nature can stir up a blizzard in the middle of May, I'd learned that pregnancy can create a storm of its own.

While I continued to grieve for my stillborn child, I longed for my womb to be expanding with life. But the conflicting feelings between my head and my heart had not yet been resolved. There was a constant murmur within me as two distinct voices—my heart and my head—whispered conflicting opinions on whether or not it was wise to try conceiving again.

My heart longed to carry another baby, to give birth, to expand our family with another living child. With its every beat, I was reminded that we had had one successful pregnancy and were raising our beautiful daughter. And my heart dared to believe in the possibility of giving her a living sibling.

But my head told me it wasn't possible, almost mocking the whispers of hope that emanated from my broken yet cautiously optimistic heart. *If God wanted you to have another child, he wouldn't have turned the previous two lives you carried to dust.* My body had failed twice, and my mind—or rather, the Enemy—preyed on its weakness. While I was not at fault for either of my losses, the battle between my head and my heart made it difficult to discern between truth and lies. *You are responsible for the death of your babies—and for the heartache of your family. Do you really want to do that to them again?* How could I even consider another pregnancy when I knew it could end up hurting not only me but also the ones I loved?

I hated what pregnancy loss had done to my family, and I hated what it had done to my heart. I hated that my attempts at family planning hadn't gone according to my plan. Pregnancy was supposed to result in raising a child, but instead it had crashed my world, bringing me to my knees. I watched families around me grow, yet mine seemed to remain stagnant. I hated that my motherhood story was steeped in grief while others seemed to be writing stories of nothing but joy.

And yet I loved the idea of having another child—expanding

our family was something both Luke and I wanted. It would take courage to do so knowing that a now uncertain path might land us in another pit of despair. While my husband was optimistic—bless his heart—that we had a good chance at a successful pregnancy, I believed the odds were against us, no matter what the statistics or doctors said. I had already lost two pregnancies and had no way of knowing if God would allow me to keep another baby. But I had a choice to make.

It wasn't just a choice about whether or not to try again; I needed to choose who I was going to listen to. I could choose to listen to the Enemy, backing down in fear and allowing him to take hold of my heart and my motherhood. Or I could choose to listen to God, embracing his words and promises and trusting him to redeem the broken parts of my motherhood—even if things didn't end the way I wanted them to.

In the midst of Satan's deceitful whispers, I had to remember that he wasn't in charge. If he had been, there was no way I would have survived the previous ten months, let alone our earlier attempt to grow our family from one child to two. It was God who had helped me through the barrenness of pregnancy loss and gripped my hand when I didn't think I could keep going. If I refused to keep living—if I gave up and allowed my heart to be bound up in insecurity and fear—I'd be just where Satan wanted me. But if I chose to put my heart on the line, to risk loss in the name of love, I'd be headed straight toward God—to a place where I would be forced to rely on him, forced to trust him, forced to accept the help that only he could offer.

Friend, it takes courage to keep going when your baby's heart has stopped. And when it comes to pregnancy after miscarriage or stillbirth, it takes courage to try again when previous attempts have, at times, made you wish your own heart had stopped. It takes courage to attempt what seems impossible—to believe that God might write a happy ending to your story of loss even when he has allowed it to be so painful. It takes courage to allow yourself to dream again when you've become so intimately acquainted with the things of nightmares. And it takes courage to give your hand to God and allow him to lead you through what could very well be a treacherous journey.

Yes, it takes courage to forge ahead when hope and healing have been in short supply; yet you have been courageous all along and accompanied by a God who hasn't left your side. In pursuing a subsequent pregnancy, you're courageously choosing to believe that God is good and that he can redeem your history of loss— even when you don't understand why it's part of your story in the first place.

Even with loss still fresh in your mind, you can find the courage to try again by leaning on the God of help. Read his promises and let them sink into your empty spaces. Slip your hand in his, and rest in the certainty that he won't let go. Walk bravely forward knowing he's walking right next to you.

God, you tell me that children are a precious gift, and, oh, how aware I am of that truth! I long to carry a precious baby in my womb. I long to give birth to a living child and raise that child in your name. But my body has become a barrier in doing so. God, as I consider another pregnancy, help me to tune out the accusatory and pessimistic voices that plague my mind. Remind me that those voices are not from you. Help me remember that you are my helper and not someone who wants to hurt me. I'm still hurting. I still long for my child who never took a breath on this earth. And I still wonder why you allowed my baby to die. Remind me that you have grasped my hand and are leading me through the shadows that mark my life. You are my help, God, in the seasons past and the seasons to come. When I am afraid of what the future holds, let me find peace in knowing that you hold me.

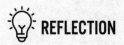

REFLECTION

In what ways has God led you during your journey toward another pregnancy? What does courage look like for you in the midst of conflicting messages between your head and your heart?

LETTER

If you could speak to your baby, what would you say about having faith and courage now in relation to the risk of what might come next?

Day 2

CHOOSING HOPE OVER DOUBT

*"For I know the plans I have for you," declares
the L*ORD*, "plans to prosper you and not to harm
you, plans to give you hope and a future."*
—JEREMIAH 29:11

Nine months after losing Micah, Luke and I decided to start trying for another baby. Shortly after making this decision, I went away for the weekend with some girlfriends, which gave my brain a slight reprieve from the constant pregnancy- and grief-related thoughts I had. Upon returning home from that trip, I was settling onto the couch to wind down when I suddenly felt sick to my stomach.

The sensation came out of nowhere, and while I briefly considered the possibility I could be pregnant, I ultimately brushed it off as my body's response to a lack of sleep and poor food choices over the course of a long weekend. After all, there was no way I could be pregnant. At least, that's what I told myself.

We had been intimate only twice, and other than an upset stomach, there was no reason to think I might be pregnant. I hadn't even missed a period yet. Plus, it was too early to be experiencing symptoms. Especially since I'd been pregnant three times without experiencing morning sickness. Surely the timing was nothing more than a coincidence.

But hidden in the deepest crevices of my heart, I hoped the feeling in my stomach was more than just the effects of a long, indulgent weekend.

I hoped it was a baby.

Luke and I had spent months deciding whether or not we would try to have another child. After experiencing two consecutive losses—an ectopic pregnancy and a stillbirth—we weren't sure we had the emotional capacity to endure another pregnancy. But we met with specialists. We prayed. We talked and talked some more. And we finally made the decision to try again.

So, try we did.

And pray I did. Not only to become pregnant but to become pregnant quickly. The expansion of our family had already taken longer than I had anticipated, and I wanted to move forward as quickly as possible. I didn't know if God had another baby in store for us, but I knew that even if he did, my definition of "quickly" differed greatly from his. After two years of loss and grief, I was convinced that his timing would never align with mine. I knew better than to assume that my plans looked anything like his.

So, that evening when my stomach began to turn, I slammed shut the doors of my heart, blocking out the idea that just maybe I had conceived more quickly than I could have imagined. It had been just ten days since we had begun trying—surely it was impossible for me to be pregnant already! I wanted to open the doors to my heart just a crack—to allow a sliver of hope, an inkling of possibility to sneak in—but I was afraid to do so. I was afraid to hope another baby was planted within my womb while I was still grieving; afraid to hope that life could thrive within me when I'd seen it wither twice. And I was afraid that if I did allow myself to hope, my heart would be broken beyond repair if another baby called my womb—but never my arms—home.

The churning of my stomach and my mind was both overwhelming and exhausting, so I turned in early that night. As I burrowed under the blankets, I buried the seed of hope that desperately wanted to sprout. I felt foolish for even thinking it might grow into something beautiful, something *alive*. After all, I'd been trudging through the desert of loss for almost two years, and the likelihood of something flourishing there seemed slim. I was afraid that if I nurtured that seed of hope at all, I would only be crushed by the realization that it would never produce life.

Looking back, I realize it wasn't just that I doubted the possibility of being pregnant; I also doubted God's goodness. I doubted his ability to bring beauty from ashes. So often during the long months of loss and grief, I wondered if God was punishing me for doing something wrong. Perhaps I was failing in my role as a mother to my living child or I was never cut out to be a mother in the first place. Perhaps I had failed some test I hadn't realized I was taking. Based on the heartache and turmoil that now played a leading role in the story of my motherhood, I doubted God had anything good left for me. And to be honest, I didn't think I deserved it. As I received news of friends and family members becoming pregnant and of babies being born, I knew his goodness was evident in the lives of others, but it seemed absent in mine.

But the doubt wasn't from God. It was a trap set by Satan. A trap that sent me stumbling into a hole of hopelessness. A trap that caused me to focus on myself and my failures instead of on God and his goodness. A trap that convinced me life would always be dark. It was all too easy for me to think that God had left me to rot in the hole and would therefore withhold all good things from my life.

It is true that our failures are many in this life, and it is true that hardship is guaranteed—whether or not it's related to motherhood. Yet, right there in the pages of Scripture, God promises that he has good plans for us regardless of our flaws and failures. He does not make plans to harm us but instead chooses to give us a reason to hope as we look forward to a future full of his goodness.

God's plan for our lives offers us hope, while Satan's plan is to convince us there is no hope. As I wondered if I could be pregnant, God was speaking hope, if only I would listen. Satan wanted me to believe no good thing could come in the morning, that the darkness of disappointment and grief would last forever. He wanted to keep me all to himself in that hole of hopelessness because he knew his best work takes place in isolation. Maybe I didn't deserve another child, but there had been countless other things in my life that were also undeserved that God, in his goodness, had granted me anyway.

> May the God of hope fill you with all joy and peace as you trust in him, so that you may overflow with hope by the power of the Holy Spirit. (Romans 15:13)

We worship the God of hope, who promises more than what those lies of Satan would have us believe. But we must be bold in keeping our hearts open to hope, while shutting out the hopelessness that only the Enemy speaks. We may not know what tomorrow holds; we aren't able to predict the future. In fact, we are promised that we will face trials and heartaches for the duration of our lives. But God also promises us a future filled with hope. Even as we walk through uncertain circumstances and fear the outcome, God will not use our experiences to harm us.

Friend, if hopelessness is part of your pregnancy-after-loss story, remember that God has good plans for you—plans that are so much better than your own. There are no guarantees in this life, even when it comes to the things God has declared as good, such as children. And while neither you nor I know the plans God has for your womb, we are guaranteed that his goodness will prevail. And because of that, there is every reason to march forward, even when what we hope for seems impossible.

God, thank you for your promise of a beautiful future, no matter how hopeless my heart is today. The sorrow I feel from losing a baby I loved so much has made it difficult for me to believe that light will ever shine in my life again. I'm scared to hope, God. Afraid that if I do, my heart won't be able to recover if the path ahead includes ongoing disappointment, heartbreak, and loss. When my circumstances seem harsh, I sink into a hole of hopelessness because I doubt your plans for me. When I am in the dark, God, remind me of your goodness, plant hope within my heart, and carry me out into your light.

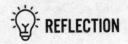

REFLECTION

In what ways is Satan stealing your hope? How has God shown you his goodness even when you doubted it?

LETTER

Describe for your child what your hope looks like in the face of what seems impossible.

Day 3

THE COURAGE TO REJOICE TODAY WITHOUT KNOWING WHAT TOMORROW HOLDS

Therefore do not worry about tomorrow, for tomorrow will worry about itself. Each day has enough trouble of its own.
—MATTHEW 6:34

My eyes flicked open and adjusted to the morning sunlight. It was the beginning of a new day, a fresh start. But the familiar feeling of nausea followed me out of bed and into the kitchen. I cracked two eggs into a frying pan but soon realized I'd be skipping breakfast—just the smell of food made my face turn green. As I plated the eggs for my daughter, Annabel, and watched her eat, I wondered if I should take a pregnancy test.

I didn't want to. I was afraid of both a negative and a positive result. A negative would cause great disappointment—grief, even—over a baby that I so desperately wanted to be there. A positive would cause panic to seep from the cracks of my already broken heart like egg whites from a cracked shell because I would question whether or not the baby would live.

My thoughts were scrambled with worry and wonder and what-ifs. My mind refused to rest. And even though my period wasn't due for another five days, the question spun frantically through my mind: *Am I pregnant?* While I would never know the answers to so many other questions I had asked over the course of the past two years, there was an easy way to determine the answer to this one.

So I dropped off Annabel at school and stopped at the drug-store to purchase a pregnancy test. Regardless of the result, I knew one wouldn't be enough to convince me, so I walked out with a box of three.

Once home, I locked myself in the bathroom, despite being home alone, and ripped open the box with shaking hands. I removed one test from its plastic wrapper, dropped my pants, and settled onto the porcelain throne. With the test stick in hand, cap removed, I held it under a stream of urine, anxiously considering what the result might be.

It felt like the bravest thing I'd ever done. Because no matter what was about to appear on that tiny plastic screen, I knew it had the potential to break my heart. If the result was negative, it might just be the first in a long series of negatives. And if the result happened to be positive, I knew it might not stay that way. A negative would at least leave nothing in question. It would be clear there was no baby to bring home. But a positive result? That would leave everything in question. Would I get to keep this baby? Would I have an ectopic pregnancy? A miscarriage? A stillbirth? Would this baby survive past the first trimester? Or the second or third? Would this baby live outside of my womb? And the only answer to any of those questions was a very unsettling "maybe."

I spent three long minutes not looking at the test window, and, mostly as a means to distract myself, I prayed. It was more of a chant, really, as I repeated, "God, help me. God, help me. God, help me." I didn't exactly know what to pray for because I was unsure of God's plan, but what I did know was that no matter the result, I would need to rely on God to help me deal with it.

When the time was up, I took a deep breath and picked up the test I'd left on the bathroom floor. One bright-pink line illuminated the test window. And next to it? Another line, though faint, confirming the test was positive.

The rhythm of my heart sped up, beating heavily against my chest. I was in disbelief. So, naturally, I took another test. And after another three minutes, the same result peered back at me through the window.

A baby was growing within me.

And yet, my emotional response was flat, lacking the enthusiasm I had, at one time, come to expect when discovering that I was expecting. In an instant, the question on my mind changed from *Am I pregnant?* to *Will I still be pregnant tomorrow?* without me fully registering the magnitude of simply being pregnant.

I was more concerned with what tomorrow would hold than with what I was holding in my womb at that very moment. As I stared at the two positive pregnancy tests, I knew that by the next day I might get a different result—I knew one of those lines could fade and the fragile life forming within me could vanish without notice. What would happen when I inevitably took the third pregnancy test that had yet to be unpackaged? Fear that this gift of life might be taken before I even had the chance to unwrap it held my head and my heart captive. Instead of rejoicing over what I knew to be true in that moment, I instantly worried about tomorrow.

Despite this exact scenario being something I had prayed for fervently for the better part of a year, the joy and excitement I had experienced at the onset of previous pregnancies wasn't there. This pregnancy was different. I knew too well that the baby in my womb might never make it home with me, even if we did spend the next nine months together.

God had opened my womb, but the immediate fear over what the days, weeks, and months ahead might hold caused distress instead of relief. I forfeited joy over a much-wanted pregnancy and instead let the thought of what might happen sweep the breath of gladness right out of my lungs.

My response wasn't out of the ordinary. It made a lot of sense, actually. Trauma during my past pregnancies had changed the landscape of my mind, and I was unable to bury the memory of loss in order to embrace the reality of life. The sting of death lingered, and I knew I had no control over it happening again.

And yet, as I sit here today, I can honestly say that I regret not allowing myself to rejoice over the presence of new life that day. It was the final time I would have the opportunity to watch the empty space of a pregnancy-test window fill with the pink signs of life—well, not counting the next day, when I took the third pregnancy test and was met with another positive result. Instead of resting in the possibility of an answered prayer, I chose to worry about a tomorrow over which I had no control anyway.

No matter what happened, God was caring for me and my unborn child, and we were both loved beyond comprehension. I wish I would have, even for a moment at a time, unwound my heart from the fear of tomorrow and allowed myself to feel joy for the presence of life that day. Because no matter how long it did or did not house itself within my womb, life in any capacity is precious. Besides, worrying would not keep my baby's life from ending—only God could do that.

Friend, I know it might seem impossible to live one day at a time—to celebrate the gift of life from day to day instead of setting your heart and mind on the uncertainty of what tomorrow might hold. You might not be there yet, and that's okay. Pregnancy after loss is incredibly hard, plain and simple—and worry is a mother's natural response to the uncertainty of what might be in store for her child's life.

Despite all the unknowns, I want to encourage you to process and rejoice over what you know to be true today. You are carrying an already-loved baby, and that is cause for joy right now—no matter what happens tomorrow.

> This is the day that the Lord has made;
> let us rejoice and be glad in it. (Psalm
> 118:24 esv)

There is no predicting the duration of your sweet baby's life. And I know how hard it is to come to a place of joy when you, as a loving mother, fear that life will end too soon. But even in the uncertainty of tomorrow, one thing is for sure: God has given you the gift of today. Your baby is here with you, right now, being carried in the sacred space of your womb with so much love.

I know it's not easy to lay fear to rest, even for just a moment, but this precious life is worth celebrating. You have this day with your baby—let your joy be greater than your fear. Take comfort in what you know to be true in this moment—that your body is carrying a much-prayed-for baby. And let tomorrow worry about itself.

It takes courage to live one day at a time, trusting God to hold tomorrow for you. He's given you today with your precious child, and even though there is a very normal flurry of emotions swirling within you, I pray that you will courageously wrap your fingers around joy and celebrate this day in hopeful anticipation of what God can do.

God, I praise and thank you for the gift of life that you have graciously placed within my womb. I love this baby so much already, but I am afraid I'm going to experience loss again. This joyous occasion has been diminished with intense anxiety because of my uncertainty over what tomorrow holds. God, help me find joy in today. I want to celebrate this precious life you have created because if today is all I have with my baby, I want it to be a good one. Allow my love for this child to be greater than my fear. And if tomorrow brings trouble, thank you for the promise of providing for all of my needs in every circumstance.

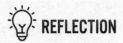

REFLECTION

What worries are stealing your peace today? Write them down. Now, think of three times when your worries never material-ized and write them down. What can you do to reclaim joy over this pregnancy today?

LETTER

Tell your baby at least three ways his or her presence is bringing you joy and why this little life is worthy of celebration.

Day 4

THE COURAGE TO SAY "I'M PREGNANT"

Rejoice with those who rejoice; mourn with those who mourn.

—Romans 12:15

You might think it would be easy telling Luke I was pregnant again. After all, he was an active participant in creating the baby I was carrying, which made it not just my baby, but *our* baby. And yet, I was nervous.

How will he react? Will he be as scared as I am? How will he respond if this baby dies too?

I worried about another pregnancy being lost due to my body's failure to nurture the small life within it. If that was the case, how could I not feel as if my husband's thrice-broken heart was my fault? It would be *my* body to blame.

But being my baby's father, and the man I loved most in this world, he deserved to know sooner rather than later. And perhaps more than that, I knew I would need his immediate support. The thought of withholding news of a new baby seemed cruel after all

21

the time he'd spent suffering right alongside me. So, I told him late in the evening, after our daughter was in bed, to ensure the news could be spoken without interruption.

I couldn't bring myself to say the words "I'm pregnant," or even to say that we were going to have a baby—something about those phrases suggested certainty, and I was anything but certain. Instead, I broke the news by saying, "I took a pregnancy test—and it was positive." That felt easier than stating there was a precious child growing within me, a treasured life over which I had no control. A baby who was here now but could be gone later.

I was surprised when my husband responded with enthusiasm.

"That's good news!" he said. "That was fast." His tone was cheerfully optimistic, a perspective I couldn't quite muster before knowing if my body would even allow this baby to continue growing.

"I think everything is going to work out this time," he said. "I just have a feeling."

But the only feeling I had was confusion. Being unsure whether my baby would make it, not just past the first trimester but the second and third as well, made it difficult to decide when to begin telling others of my pregnancy. I could no longer rely on the conventional wisdom that it is safe to announce a pregnancy upon reaching the second trimester. No, I knew that it is never truly safe to announce a pregnancy—there is always a chance of having to retract your statement.

I vowed not to tell anyone else until I had at least heard my baby's heartbeat. An official pregnancy announcement would set the expectation that I would bring home a baby, and I couldn't promise to do so. I was afraid if I told others too soon—and by too soon, I mean anytime before my baby was safely in my arms—I'd have to make tearful phone calls saying, "Never mind; there is no baby," through uncontrollable gasps and incoherent speech. These were the bad news calls that made me feel like a failure, an embarrassment to my family. And they were calls I knew all too well.

But God had different plans.

Ten days after that conversation with my husband, I also told two friends of my pregnancy through interactions I'm certain were divinely appointed. The truth is, I had been desperate to share the news. Desperate to speak my fears aloud. Desperate to hear words of encouragement. Desperate to unload some of the emotional weight of my pregnancy onto the shoulders of another. But I couldn't bring myself to initiate.

During my season of loss, one particular friend had walked with me through the valley of grief. She knew my hurt. She'd seen my face contort as I ugly-cried on her couch more than once. She'd taken care of my daughter on several occasions as we were dealing with visits to the ER and then the cemetery. And when I became pregnant again, my heart wanted to pour out its boiling emotions to her, knowing she could take the heat and respond with compassion.

But I was afraid. Scared that if I acknowledged my pregnancy, I would become attached to a child I didn't know if I'd get to keep. I thought that by keeping quiet I could control grief's ability to take over my heart should this baby not have the opportunity to live outside my body. But I was wrong—that kind of self-protection doesn't exist. In the case of loss, I would be devastated whether or not I allowed myself to be vulnerable. What I really needed was support.

At the time, my friend was overwhelmed with her own high-risk pregnancy as well as the demands of mothering two young children. As it often goes with the busyness of motherhood, we hadn't spoken in a while. But I told myself that if she just so happened to call, I'd open the vault and invite her in.

Well, God initiated that conversation for me.

At a moment when I had the house to myself, my phone rang, and my friend's name jumped off the screen in bold letters. After she updated me on the circumstances surrounding her difficult pregnancy, it was time for me to speak.

"I wasn't going to tell anyone this, but I think God wants me to tell you," I said.

"Oh," she whispered, her voice suddenly sober with concern.

"I'm pregnant. And I'm scared."

I forced the words out of my mouth quickly so I wouldn't have the chance to change my mind. She congratulated me, which I expected, but she also offered words of comfort and validation. She empathized, as her own experiences with pregnancy hadn't been all that smooth. I cried with relief at feeling less alone. It was good to have a shoulder to cry on.

Later that evening, I met another friend for dinner. It had been months since we'd seen each other, which meant there would be lots of catching up to do. She didn't waste any time informing me that she was pregnant with her second child after enduring an emergency situation with her first pregnancy that landed her baby in the NICU for several weeks. She, too, was treading through the murky waters of a high-risk pregnancy, and I knew I could trust her with my news. Again, I was met with empathy, compassion, and words that spoke hope into my heart. God knew I needed companions to ease the emotional burdens I was carrying, and he put two people in my path that day who could shoulder some of that weight with me.

A few weeks later, I was spending Christmas vacation under one big roof with my entire family. I had decided to keep the news of my pregnancy to myself. I didn't want my family to spend the holiday worrying about me or my baby, nor did I want to be the center of attention. I especially didn't want to plant the seed in their hearts of another grandchild, niece, nephew, or cousin joining the family, knowing this baby might not survive.

By withholding the news, I felt that I was protecting not just myself but them also. I could avoid the awkward vulnerability of openly discussing my physical and emotional state, and they could avoid another potential stressor during the holiday season.

But you know what? I regret not telling them. Because it would have helped to explain my extreme emotions—the yelling, snapping, crying, and withdrawal. And it might have explained why I went home earlier than planned. They understood I was grieving for the baby I'd lost earlier that year. But that was only a portion of my reality. To fully understand my emotional state, they would have needed to know I was pregnant again and very afraid.

By withholding the news, I didn't give my family the opportunity to love me by offering support. Nor did they have the chance to celebrate my unborn baby's life that Christmas—what if that was the only chance they had?

As you consider when and how to announce your pregnancy, as well as with whom to share the news, think of the people in your life who have been supportive during seasons of loss. Who has mourned with you? Maybe it's friends and family. Maybe it's a church community or coworkers. Might you allow them to rejoice with you over this new pregnancy?

It's no doubt scary to announce the presence of a life you aren't sure will survive, but God has placed people in your life to rejoice in this new creation with you, especially when you find it difficult to rejoice yourself. Might you allow others to hold your hand as you navigate this strenuous journey? Might you give them the chance to express joy for this new life when you cannot?

You weren't made to do life alone. Take a chance. Believe that God placed people in your life to walk with you through times of mourning as well as times of rejoicing. There is no need to announce your pregnancy to the whole world—unless, of course, you want to. You don't have to plaster the news all over social media. But perhaps there are a few people you might consider giving the opportunity to support you through this joyous and daunting circumstance.

This is your pregnancy—and your heart on the line. There are no rules demanding that you announce your pregnancy at a certain time or in a certain way. Therefore, you get to decide how and when you allow others into your experience. If you choose to keep the news to yourself for a while, take heart in knowing that God is rejoicing in this new life with you, just as he mourned the life of the baby to whom you said goodbye. After all, God creates every human life with his very hands, and we know that his love for the people he has created is greater than anything else.

I know how hard it is to let others in, but may I suggest that the extra support that comes from speaking the truth of your pregnancy aloud might be just what your heart needs? Your baby deserves to be rejoiced over, and you deserve to be supported, not only by the God who loves you both but by the community in which he placed you. And while it might take an extra dose of courage to say, "I'm pregnant," how awesome will it be to have a few other people rallying around and praying for you and your baby?

You've opened your heart to your baby. Now consider opening up to others so that they can love *you* in the days and weeks to come.

God, thank you for being an ever-present support throughout the course of my pregnancy. I am afraid to announce this pregnancy to those around me because I don't want to have to make those dreaded phone calls if my baby doesn't survive. I don't want to be a source of disappointment for my family and friends. God, I ask that you point me to a few gentle souls I can trust with my heart. Give me the courage to unveil the truth about my circumstances. And if I cannot speak aloud the words "I'm pregnant," let my heart be comforted in knowing that you are rejoicing over this new life.

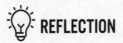 **REFLECTION**

Write down the names of two or more people (other than your husband) who possess the qualities of a trustworthy friend—people who are gentle, compassionate, and open to vulnerability. How might you allow these people to support you during your pregnancy? Write down what you need from them, and practice telling them.

 LETTER

Tell your baby about all the people you want him or her to meet. Describe how you would like to announce your pregnancy to these people.

27

Day 5

IMAGINING A DIFFERENT ENDING WHEN HISTORY BEGINS TO REPEAT ITSELF

See, I am doing a new thing!
Now it springs up; do you not perceive it?
I am making a way in the wilderness
and streams in the wasteland.

—ISAIAH 43:19

I was less than one week into the second trimester of my pregnancy when I was sent home from a prenatal appointment with a prescription for bed rest. After a surprise ultrasound and a sonographer who told me nothing about her findings, I was instructed to wait for my midwife to speak with me privately.

This wasn't the first time I'd peeled my bare body off an exam table, my mind abuzz with more questions than answers. From experience, I had learned that when a sonographer is too quiet and

29

the mood in the room is more somber than celebratory, something on the screen displays a painful truth.

As I waited impatiently, I could feel my heart sinking into a great chasm of doom, defeat rapidly coursing through my veins. I began steeling myself for the phone calls I'd have to make, the messages I'd have to send, the tears and awkward silences that filled me with a sense of dread.

How can I be here again?

It was January, a month I would forever associate with loss. Exactly one year prior, I had said goodbye to Micah in a cold, sterile hospital room, his tiny, twenty-week-old body still, the air quiet. And a year before that, I had said goodbye to Baby A, who died before being named. The past two years had begun with the loss of a baby, and the ultrasound images from those short lives were seared into my mind. One was of a baby I would never see in person, and the other of a baby with whom I would come face-to-face only after his heart had stopped.

Is this baby destined for the same fate—death before birth?

As I scanned the image on the monitor, watching intently for signs of life or death, I concluded that another loss was likely. Based on the uneasiness that hung in the air of that dimly lit room, it seemed I was in the midst of another January that would end with the weight of loss heavy on my already weary shoulders; another year that would begin with the precious life of my very own flesh and blood coming to an end.

I sat in the glow of the black-and-white screen, images from the past two years reeling through my mind. Positive pregnancy tests. Emergency room visits. Hospital stays. And no baby to bring home. I recalled the tears and groaning. The hours—days, even— curled up in bed or heaped on the floor. As much as I wanted to imagine bringing home the baby I'd just seen, knowledge of both past and present circumstances seemed to scream, *Why bother?*

When my midwife knocked on the door, I braced myself for words I expected to break my heart for a third time.

As suspected, the news wasn't good. She informed me my cervix was already thinning, which meant the wheels were already in motion for labor to begin far too early. I was told to go home and stay in bed until I could see a maternal-fetal medicine (MFM) specialist the following day. My midwife hoped that by keeping pressure off my cervix as much as possible, my body would be better equipped to continue carrying my growing baby until a specialist could confirm the findings and determine how best to proceed.

The news was expected and unexpected all at once. After experiencing loss twice before, I didn't fully believe another pregnancy could be successful. In fact, I hardly believed it at all. Yet, a small part of me clung to the belief that another loss couldn't possibly happen because surely God wouldn't allow me to suffer more than I already had.

Or would he?

Based on the information I'd been given, it appeared my pregnancy was being written in the language of the same old story. Grief. Trauma. Death. And the unique emptiness that comes only from the loss of a baby. It felt as if my mama heart was destined to forever wander in the wilderness of grief and the arid land of loss.

I shuffled through the halls of the medical complex out to my car and called my husband. As I croaked out the words "cervix thinning" and "bed rest" and asked him to come home to care for our daughter, I felt like I was choking. The air was suddenly dry, and I wondered how I would manage to drag myself through the suffocating terrain of another loss.

For thirty-some hours, I was confined to my bed, allowed to get up only to use the bathroom. Propped up against a hedge of pillows, I vacillated between self-pity and prayer. *Why me? Why this—again? God, protect my womb; protect my baby; carry us safely through this trial.* My thoughts spun around and around, demanding to know why and crying out for help.

I wanted so badly to imagine a good outcome for my baby, a different ending for the pregnancy that had been preceded by two losses. But with a cervix threatening to give out twenty-six weeks too early, I felt foolish for even entertaining that idea.

Perhaps being confined to bed was a call to rely on God's promises instead of human knowledge, to be still and allow the Lord to fight this battle for me, just as he had done for the ancient Israelites (Exodus 14:14). But waiting isn't exactly my favorite thing to do, so I tried to control the situation. I wanted so desperately to secure my baby's place in my arms, not just in my heart. So I called the specialist's office and requested an earlier appointment. I was denied and forced to wait for the appointment time that I had been assigned.

As the minutes ticked by, thoughts of all that could go wrong percolated in my mind. The idea of burying another baby caused my fear to grow exponentially. I was certain that history was repeating itself and I could do nothing to stop it.

I had mentally prepared myself for the inevitability of the bad news I would receive at my appointment with the MFM specialist the following day. And yet, when I arrived, it turned out I wasn't at all prepared for what she told me.

"Your cervix is long and strong," she stated with confidence. "It looks perfect!"

She went on to say that my midwife must have misinterpreted the previous ultrasound due to poor image quality.

I had spent more than a day expecting the worst only to discover there hadn't been a problem in the first place—it was a simple, albeit frightening, mistake. It was the first of several different-than-expected outcomes during my pregnancy.

And it was the first time I truly understood that the past does not have the authority to rule the present or the future. Nor do I. Only God does. I couldn't control how my pregnancy unfolded, but I could control my response to the way it played out. I could allow myself to flail in a sea of what-ifs and drown in a pool of despair each time a concern arose, or I could march forward and hope for the best, fully accepting that my human mind holds no knowledge of tomorrow.

Yes, my history of loss played heavily into my emotional state going into another pregnancy. How could it not? I was still grieving. I was still longing for another baby to fill my arms. I was still scarred by the trauma surrounding my last two pregnancies.

But just because I had wandered in the wilderness of grief did not mean God would never lead me in a new direction. Just because my faith had been weakened in that barren land of loss did not mean God had lost the ability to quench the thirst of my parched heart and soul. And just because the road was littered with obstacles did not mean I wouldn't reach the finish line with a baby to mark the journey I'd been on.

Friend, in the face of trouble, I chose to cower in that familiar place of darkness instead of courageously seeking God's light. I chose to imagine the worst, to base my feelings on the past, and to fear the future instead of taking a chance on believing that God was leading me in a new direction and that his plans were bigger than my fears.

While I don't know how your pregnancy is playing out right now, I have no doubt that the past is likely playing a major role in how you perceive it. That's normal. You won't forget your past pregnancy or the baby you loved so dearly. And you don't have to.

But when you are convinced that history is going to repeat itself in all the worst ways, remember that this is a new pregnancy, a new baby, a new path. And while neither you nor I know what awaits at the end of it, don't allow the things that are behind you to steal your hope in the possibility of what lies ahead.

God promises to make a way where there isn't one. And while there is no telling exactly what this might mean for your future or your family, trust him to lead you out of the wilderness of grief and loss.

As you look back on the hurt and heartache of the past, remember to enjoy your present. And try with all your might to remember that a beautiful future is often born from a difficult past.

God, I am so deeply afraid that history is going to repeat itself. That this pregnancy will end prematurely and that my arms will once again be left empty. Remind me that my past does not dictate my future and that even in the worst-case scenario, you are doing a new thing that will eventually be used for my good. Remind me how you have already been faithful in leading me through the wilderness, how you have watered my soul even when grief and hopelessness have dried it up. God, help me to not get so caught up in the past that I miss the beauty of the present.

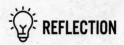

REFLECTION

In what ways are the losses of the past affecting your current pregnancy? How do you see God making a way for you in the wilderness?

LETTER

Share with your baby your hopes about how your pregnancy will be completed.

Day 6

THE COURAGE TO STAY GROUNDED
WHEN STORM CLOUDS HOVER

God is our refuge and strength,
*   an ever-present help in trouble.*
Therefore we will not fear, though the earth give
*   way*
*   and the mountains fall into the heart of the*
*   sea,*
though its waters roar and foam
*   and the mountains quake with their*
*   surging.*

—Psalm 46:1–3

It had been two weeks since the cervix scare, and while I hadn't fully recovered from the panic of that experience, my cervix had continued to present as long and strong. The threat of losing what we had just discovered to be a baby boy seemed to be

37

passing, or at least diminishing. I was slowly starting to believe that maybe my body was equipped to carry this baby for a full nine months—or at least to the point where he would have a chance at survival.

I was fortunate to have the gift of weekly prenatal appointments. During these appointments I was able to hear the reassuring sound of my baby's heart filling the room with a steady and strong beat. I saw his growing limbs on the ultrasound screen, bouncing against the walls of my womb, even though I could not yet feel them. I saw his beating heart dance in the darkness. And I praised God for these wonderful signs of life. These sights and sounds provided me with a glimmer of hope, and I left these appointments with a sense of peace, knowing that all was well and that I'd only have to wait another week to see and hear him again.

Such appointments were the highlight of a pregnancy that was progressing in the shadow of loss. And the ultrasounds—the only evidence I had that my baby was alive and kicking—were quite literally a light in the darkness. I lay in that dark room mesmerized by the images that shone from the screen. With each positive report, I was filled with the hope that I was moving further and further from the storm of pregnancy loss. And I thought maybe I was finally stepping out from under the looming clouds of grief and the rain of tears.

It was at one such appointment that my doctor commented on how beautiful my cervix looked. She said she was glad to see that the weight of my growing baby was not having any effect on its ability to stay put. I took a moment to savor the information, to let the good news of another positive appointment sink into my bones.

But there was more news that day, and it wasn't so good. After measuring my cervix, my doctor directed my attention to a dark shadow that resembled nothing more than a shapeless blob. It seemed harmless to me, but she explained that it was something called "amniotic sludge," and that, while she could not predict how it would affect my pregnancy, it was known to cause preterm labor. (Much to my dismay, it would continue to show itself on ultrasounds throughout my pregnancy.) That term "amniotic sludge" sounded like something from a sci-fi movie, but it was a scene that could have been taken straight from a horror movie that flashed through my mind.

I saw the face of tiny Micah, who had been a victim of preterm premature rupture of membranes (PPROM), lying still, unbreathing, and cradled in the palms of my hands. My mind replayed the cries of babies coming from other rooms of the labor and delivery unit while I'd sat in my quiet room, staring at my dead baby. And of course, I remembered leaving the hospital with nothing more than a teddy bear. To me, preterm labor was equivalent to death, and I was immediately reminded that the storm clouds were still looming. For all I knew, loss was still on the horizon.

I suddenly felt weak, both physically and emotionally. Just moments before, when I'd heard what I wanted to hear and seen what I wanted to see, I had felt confident, strong. My pregnancy was heading in the right direction—toward life instead of loss. But my confidence crumbled at the first sign of trouble.

I went home to search for more information about the mysterious sludge my doctor had pointed out. Every report I read confirmed that it was indeed a risk factor for preterm labor. And with that, the storm clouds got a little darker and a lot scarier. I was already at high risk, and all I could do now was melt into the couch and wait for the rain to start falling.

The peace that had swept over my body at hearing my baby's heartbeat and seeing the bright outline of his body that day disappeared when I received that little bit of unexpected news. And again, I was afraid.

For many women, pregnancy is a time of great hope, as it should be. And maybe even quiet contentment as they imagine soon stepping into the future of their dreams. But it's more complicated for those of us who have experienced loss. In some ways, the feeling of a baby in our arms is so close that we can taste the sweet morsels of anticipation. But in many ways, the idea that we will ever get to carry our babies outside our bodies seems impossible. And the anticipation turns sour.

We long for solid ground that promises an easy path to a problem-free pregnancy, one that will definitely conclude with a healthy baby. But we also know that there is no such thing as a guaranteed happy ending. Not in this world. There is no keeping the rain from seeping into the cracks of the earth on which we stand, turning it to mush. There's no stopping the ground from shaking or the rain from falling in any aspect of our lives, really. We've been damaged, broken apart by the heartache that accompanies life in a storm-tossed world.

Yet, we still hope. Because it's the only way to survive the sometimes-unbearable conditions of this world. We cling to faith when we've got nothing else to hold on to—and sometimes I think that's the whole point of all this uncertainty and hurt.

Maybe you are in a place where optimism regarding your current pregnancy has vanished, blown away by the whipping winds of an impending storm. Maybe you've gotten some frightening news or are at a place where your pregnancy isn't progressing as smoothly as you hoped.

Instead of allowing the storm to knock you off your feet when the ground shakes, invite God into the storm with you. Let him hold you up when hardships threaten your body, mind, and even your baby. He promises to stand right next to you, no matter how strong the wind and heavy the rain. There is not one thing in this world more powerful than God, and with him, even the most difficult pregnancy can't take you down. Not in the long run, anyway. Because, yes, you've already been brought to your knees, but look at how he's pulled you back up. You're standing again, something you once thought impossible.

Even in the eye of the storm, anchor your faith in God because he's the one in control—not your circumstances. Rely on him to carry you through the torrents, and watch as his strength sweeps away your fears. You may not be capable of withstanding the storm, but God is. And he promises to steady you when the ground beneath you trembles and your knees begin to shake.

God, I so desperately want the storm of loss to be over. In fact, I wish I had never had to experience it in the first place. I'm not sure I can endure a pregnancy in which the storm clouds hover and threaten. When I receive difficult news, I become weak and begin to fear the future. Instead of hiding in fear, help me to come to you so that you can shelter me with your strength and loving presence. When I am afraid, remind me of the dark places you have already carried me through, the threats from which you have already saved me. Help me to let go of fear so I can anchor my faith in you.

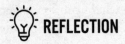

REFLECTION

How have you seen God's strength revealed during this pregnancy?

LETTER

Talk to your baby about how your pregnancy is progressing. Describe how faith is helping you to weather the possibility of another storm.

Day 7

BOLDLY PUTTING ON THE ARMOR OF GOD

Finally, be strong in the Lord and in his mighty
power. Put on the full armor of God, so that you can
take your stand against the devil's schemes.
—Ephesians 6:10–11

I was newly pregnant when I attended a church Bible study that caused me to question what my husband and I had been thinking when we decided to try for another baby. What was I thinking when I chose to believe that another pregnancy might turn out differently?

Taking a seat next to me was a woman I'd not met before whose kind eyes and magnetic smile immediately put me at ease—that is, until we started chatting and the typical small-talk questions hit me like arrows intended to rip my heart to shreds.

"Do you have kids? How many? Just one? Are you going to have more?"

I offered one-word answers while trying to keep my breathing steady and my lips from quivering.

With a sparkle in her eye and a calm smile, she went on to tell me about her young son and the early stages of her current pregnancy. I considered sharing that I, too, was pregnant again, but unlike the joy that shone on her face as she discussed her pregnancy, I knew I'd end up in tears if I described mine. Where she seemed at peace, I was conflicted. The details of my own pregnancy were too complicated to discuss without becoming emotional, so I stayed tight-lipped and awkwardly waited for the study to begin.

At some point during the sixty-minute study, the leader began discussing how to ensure the decisions we make are godly ones.

"We know our decisions are aligned with God's plans when we feel the peace that surpasses all understanding," she explained.

And I unraveled.

For months, I'd prayed for wisdom about the possibility of having another baby. I'd repeatedly asked God to make clear if and when we should start the process of trying again. I prayed that he not even allow another pregnancy if it would lead to the loss of another baby. Over time, armed with information and as much wisdom as we'd ever have when it came to the ifs and whens of a theoretical pregnancy, Luke and I pressed forward and soon found ourselves in the unknown of pregnancy after loss for a second time.

The voice of the study leader faded as the voice in my head began to shout, unheard by everyone but me. *See? You shouldn't have gotten pregnant again! You don't have the peace you're supposed to have, which means you aren't really supposed to be pregnant!*

We'd made the decision to try again, which resulted in the baby I was now carrying. But I didn't have the peace that surpassed all understanding, the very thing the study leader had said was the mark of God's will. In fact, I didn't feel much peace at all.

I suddenly felt afraid and started to panic, my breath becoming shallow. I wondered if I might lose my baby right then and there as I considered the possibility that my lack of peace might signify that my pregnancy was not aligned with God's plans.

As soon as the closing prayer was finished, I hurried to my car and began frantically scribbling a prayer of sorts inside my notebook, filling the pages with garbled questions and nonsensical though strangely realistic fears. Tears dripped onto the lined paper, causing the lines to thicken and smearing the dark ink as I cried out to God, wondering if I'd gotten it all wrong. *If I don't have that enviable peace, is my pregnancy in conflict with God's will?*

This was just the beginning of many battles that would take place over the next several months. Every time a new concern arose, I wondered if it was because I'd made the wrong decision in choosing to try for another baby. In fact, there didn't even have to be any out-of-the-ordinary concerns for my mind to spin out unanswerable questions. *Is this pregnancy actually part of God's plan? Are we wrong to try to grow our family by one? Is this all just a big mistake?* Sure, there were some moments of peace, but I can't say that such peace was constant or that it surpassed all understanding.

The message during Bible study that day may have been a biblical one, but in this battle between life and loss—this battle for hope, faith, and new life—it wasn't beneath Satan to use a biblical message to cause my knowledge of truth to scatter like leaves in the wind.

Every day, I was afraid. Grief and guilt clung to me like a wet T-shirt. The fabric of each day was riven with uncertainty and unanswered questions. From morning until night, I wrestled through trenches of deep and unsettling emotion, wondering why I'd chosen to fight this battle in the first place. Fear breezed through the flimsy shield of hope that I carried because no matter how hard I fought for my baby, I knew I wasn't guaranteed a win.

In my quest to make sense of everything, I lost sight of who and what I was actually battling against.

I wasn't in conflict with God. I was in conflict with a fractured world that had failed me and would no doubt fail me again. I was in conflict with Satan. I was in conflict with the ways he'd found to condemn me and the life inside me. He knew my weak spots and the brokenness I'd experienced. And honestly, I was in conflict with myself, with my own body and mind, as I tried to maintain a sense of control when everything was truly beyond my ability to control or comprehend.

I didn't have the power to bring the life of my baby into existence, just as I didn't have the power to keep it in existence, even by following all the recommendations and precautions. My husband and I could have tried all we wanted, but the ultimate decision to create life was out of our hands. My behavior, my feelings—they didn't hold one bit of power over God, his will, and his decisions for my life.

Friend, I have no doubt that there have been times during your pregnancy that have felt like an attack. Satan wants us to live life based only on what we can see—which is a whole lot of hurt and heartache. He wants to twist well-intentioned words and fling them at us with condemnation. He wants us to believe we're in the trenches alone, suffering because maybe, just maybe, we made the wrong choice. He wants us to think that because carrying this baby is so incredibly difficult, God must not care.

But God wants us to live by faith, not by sight (2 Corinthians

5:7). There is always more to the story than the brokenness that's so often front and center in this life. He wants us to rest in his Word and the promise that there is no condemnation for those who walk with him (Romans 8:1). He wants us to trust that he is always near. And he wants us to cling to the truth that he created this baby. *Of course he cares about the life knit together by his very own hands!*

Pregnancy after loss is hard because we *are* walking in the valley of the shadow of death—that of a beloved baby who is no longer with us. And in the darkness it's hard to hear clearly when the resounding echoes of loss and uncertainty surround us.

But we can arm ourselves with truth. We can move forward in faith, even if it means crawling and getting scraped and bruised along the way. We can put on the full armor of God, trusting in his love to guide us when the attacks threaten to overwhelm our entire being.

> The Lord your God is with you,
> > the Mighty Warrior who saves.
> He will take great delight in you. (Zephaniah 3:17)

Satan delights in seeking to harm you. God simply delights in you—and in your baby—for you both are part of his glorious creation. Arm yourself with that truth the next time you hear the whispers questioning whether this pregnancy was actually God's plan. You can silence them by remembering that every life is created by God.

God, there are so many mixed messages swirling around me, and I struggle to interpret them. I wonder what your will is, and sometimes I still wonder if I did something to cause my loss or if it's my fault that pregnancy after loss is so hard. I want certainty, God. I want answers. I want the theme of my pregnancy to be hope, but there are just so many darn arrows flying at me, so many attacks from the world and the Evil One. I want a peace that surpasses all understanding, but if I don't get it, arm me with truth. Remind me that you love me and my baby. Show me that you delight in us. Help me to cling to your words and to look to you for hope. Guide me through the attacks that threaten my peace, and help me to trust that you are in control.

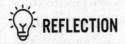 **REFLECTION**

What battles are you fighting as you progress through pregnancy? Read through the description of the armor of God in Ephesians 6:13–17. Which piece of armor do you need most right now?

 LETTER

God delights in your baby—and so do you! Tell your baby all the reasons you know this to be true.

Day 8

THE COURAGE TO ENDURE
THE LONG, HARD WAIT

See how the farmer waits for the land to yield its valuable crop, patiently waiting for the autumn and spring rains.

—JAMES 5:7

I don't want to be here!" I sobbed as my mom wrapped her arms around me in a quiet nook of a bustling house. It was Christmas—but Christmas without Micah—and I was struggling to celebrate much of anything. While my mom attempted to comfort me in my grief, she was unaware of the additional stress weighing on me because she was unaware of the baby I was carrying. I had *wanted* to want to be with my family during the holiday season, but now the only thing I truly wanted was to drive the six hours back to my own home.

The house was buzzing with life, the noise level perpetually escalating with the combined voices of five young children who bounced around wildly. I wanted to channel some of their enthusiasm, but the cacophony served only to remind me of the one voice that was missing—Micah's. He had been born earlier that year but was not celebrating with us.

The sheer abundance of life bursting at the seams of that house should have been a welcome distraction from the resounding grief that was so difficult to silence; from the anxiety surrounding the whisper of life in my womb; from the longing for my reality to be different. But no matter how much life was swirling around me, I was fixated on the life that had come to an end. A child was missing from my arms, and I was afraid that another would soon go missing from my womb.

It wasn't just that I didn't want to be far away from the comfort of my own home. It was also that I didn't want to be there as the token grieving person whose unpredictable emotions made people uncomfortable. I didn't want to be there as the woman who had lost a baby. I didn't want to be there in a place where grief and anxiety bound together my loss and pregnancy after losing Micah. I didn't want to be there as the secretly pregnant woman who was frantic with worry that the baby I was carrying could die, and that it could happen in that house, with an audience.

But mostly I didn't want to be there amid the waiting. The waiting to see if and how my pregnancy would progress. The waiting to rise out of the depths of grief. The waiting for my baby.

Waiting for those things was hard enough, but what made it even more challenging was that in some twisted way, I was also waiting for tragedy to bring an end to the waiting altogether. I was waiting for *something* to happen, and I knew whatever that something was could be devastating as much as it could be incredible.

I wanted to be there with a baby already in my arms—not waiting for the baby I was carrying to maybe, hopefully, one day make it safely into my embrace. Being stuck in the wait was *not* where I wanted to be. No, I wanted to skip straight from the positive pregnancy test to the full-term birth of my crying baby, with no time between for questioning what may or may not happen.

I would have given anything for a time machine that could transport me from positive pregnancy test straight to the delivery room echoing with shouts of congratulations. The wait would have been so much easier if I could have escaped it altogether. If I never actually had to travel the long stretch of time between implantation and the moment my body yielded a beautiful, healthy baby—that is, if we both made it that far.

But that was nothing more than wishful thinking. Because time machines aren't real, and wombs were designed to grow babies slowly. It wasn't lost on me that the combination of time and growth were necessary ingredients for creating the sweetest possible outcome for my baby and for my heart. But that knowledge didn't stop me from wishing I were on the other side of the unknowing.

Because not knowing what's going to happen is the hardest part of waiting, isn't it?

Had I known for certain that my baby boy would make it out of my womb alive, the waiting would have been more than bearable; in fact, it would have been enjoyable. I would have gleefully planned for my son's arrival by stocking the closet with tiny clothes, painting the nursery, purchasing baby gear, and assembling the crib.

But as a mama who was expecting a baby without fully expecting it to live, the wait was extremely hard and the months excruciatingly long. Not all pregnancies are created equal. The pregnancy that occurs after losing a baby stretches into the slowest-moving weeks and months of a woman's life. I like to say that my pregnancy felt like it was eighteen months long—twice as long as a normal pregnancy—and sometimes I believe that it actually was. The better part of a year is a long time to wait for anything, especially in our life-on-demand world. But there is no longer wait, no longer *pregnancy*, than the one that comes after losing a baby.

I waited and waited and waited for my body to produce a baby while, at the same time, waiting to find out if it would be another dry year in which I would endure another loss. The seed of life was planted, and now I had no choice but to wait and see if it thrived. It was the ultimate test of patience, and while I won't pretend I handled it gracefully, I handled it nonetheless. Because, like the farmer who waits for the land to produce crops, what else could I do?

Friend, I can only imagine that you, too, are muddling through the long, hard wait. Maybe you're wondering if all the hard work you've put in will pay off. Or if all the energy you've expended will ultimately bring your baby home.

Waiting for your baby to make the transition from your womb to your arms is anything but easy. I can almost hear you groaning, knowing the wait is necessary but resenting it. But good things take time and also courage when you aren't sure how the season of waiting will end.

> I believe that I shall look upon the goodness of the
>> LORD
>> in the land of the living!
> Wait for the LORD;
>> be strong, and let your heart take courage;
>> wait for the LORD! (Psalm 27:13–14 ESV)

In the days ahead, there may be plenty of times you'll wish the wait were over, but know this: God uses waiting seasons to produce not only fruits of the Spirit but also the fruits of your labor. And in the case of pregnancy after loss, the labor, the hard and grueling work, takes place well before stepping into the labor and delivery room. On the hard days, remember that you are another day closer to reaping what your body has worked so hard to grow—a baby.

While there are many things we can't know on this side of the waiting, one thing we can know for sure is that this season won't be wasted. God produces goodness—that baby inside of you being a sure sign of it—no matter how messy the wait or what the outcome may be.

Just as farmers water crops they can't yet see during their season of waiting, you're nourishing your baby, waiting for him or her to grow strong enough to safely emerge from your womb. It might not seem ideal, but there is life to be found even in the waiting as your baby slowly moves toward the good and proper time to be born.

As you wait for your baby, for the hurt to end and the healing to take place, wait on the Lord, for he is good. Even in the long, treacherous unknowing.

God, I feel stuck in what seems like the longest, most difficult wait of my life. No matter how many days of this pregnancy are behind me, I feel like I'm never going to reach the finish line. I wonder if I'll ever get to hold my baby. I wish for time to rush by so I won't have to endure such a long period of not knowing what to expect. I might not like it, but I know you designed pregnancy to be a slow process to form every detail of my precious baby.

God, through loss I've experienced what feels like a motherhood drought. And I want so desperately to be in a season of abundance and thriving. I pray that as I nourish my body and my baby, you, too, will nourish these things, along with my heart. I pray that you will grow this baby into a healthy little human and allow me to reap this life that has been sown within me. As I wait for my baby, help me to wait patiently on you and your timing. Remind me of your goodness when my patience wears thin.

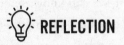

REFLECTION

Pregnancy after loss is a season of waiting—for a positive pregnancy test, the sound of a heartbeat, updates from medical providers, and, of course, the birth of your baby. What are you waiting for right now? A year from now, when you are on the other side of the unknowing, what would you like to be able to say about how you navigated this season of waiting?

LETTER

Challenge yourself to name at least three good things this season of waiting has produced in you, such as various fruits of the Spirit (Galatians 5:22–23). Share them in a letter to your baby.

Day 9

THE COURAGE TO CHOOSE A NEW MEDICAL TEAM

*If any of you lacks wisdom, you should ask
God, who gives generously to all without
finding fault, and it will be given to you.*

—James 1:5

It was intuition that drove me to the ER at seventeen weeks pregnant with Micah and parked my increasingly unreliable body in the hospital bed.

Something was off, though there weren't yet any obvious signs of danger. What I knew wasn't much—only that I hadn't been able to get out of bed for two days due to vague symptoms including dizziness and changes in vision—but it was enough to know I hadn't experienced anything like this before. It was enough for me to understand that something was wrong.

The doctor didn't have much to go on other than the

ambiguous symptoms I described, but he did observe me for a short time before ultimately assuring me that both my baby and I appeared to be healthy and thriving.

I wasn't confident in the doctor's findings, but the sound of my baby's heartbeat had brought me a sense of comfort, and I left the hospital feeling grateful for that.

But a short time later, I began bleeding.

Paralyzed at first by the sight of blood, and knowing it could be a sign of a serious problem, I talked myself through some deep-breathing exercises before telling my husband. He hovered near the dining room table, where I was speaking on the phone with a nurse, waiting for advice on how to proceed. After detailing how much blood I was seeing and how often I was seeing it, she instructed me to keep an eye on things overnight and speak with my doctor in the morning.

I did just that and once again landed in the ER, where I was again told that everything was okay. That my baby was well. That the doctor didn't see enough blood to be concerned, despite my insistence that there had been much more blood in the previous twenty-four hours than what he was seeing at that exact moment.

The doctor assured me that my pregnancy was progressing normally and began processing my release.

"I feel better now, don't you?" Luke said after the doctor left the room.

"No," I responded as I tugged my yoga pants up over my baby bump. "I know something is wrong."

Something was indeed wrong, and less than twenty-four hours later my concerns were substantiated when my water broke. At just under eighteen weeks pregnant, this nightmarish development sent my pregnancy into a drama that ended with the stillbirth of my baby.

While my body had been whispering trouble for days, making it difficult for medical professionals to detect a problem, my mother's intuition had spoken loud and clear. Before the bright-red blood made its appearance, my intuition had waved a red flag, alerting me that my baby was in danger. Even without tangible proof—even without confirmation from professionals or experts— sometimes a mother just knows.

The same intuition played a major role in my decision to change medical providers during my pregnancy after two losses.

I had been with my ob-gyn for over a decade when I became pregnant after loss for the second time. She had been my provider for almost the entirety of my first pregnancy and had seen me through the two losses that followed. She was not just aware of my medical history but had also experienced much of it with me. She was there when we discovered that my second pregnancy was not viable due to the implanting of the fertilized egg outside my uterus. She was there for the multiple visits to her office and the ER as I staggered through my failing third pregnancy, waiting for the inevitable loss of my unborn baby. She was there when Micah was stillborn. And she was there in her office when I broke down crying two weeks later.

While she had been compassionate during the trials involved in growing our family, I sensed a need for change during our consultations about the possibility of another pregnancy. I had undeniable concerns regarding the adequacy of my cervix and my history of infection as well as multitudes of unanswered questions surrounding my losses that deserved consideration.

I had done my research and consulted with specialists from

three different practices, including one who lived and practiced out of state. They all agreed that precautions should be taken in the event that I became pregnant again. They agreed that a higher level of care would be appropriate, even necessary. They agreed that certain medications would be beneficial. They agreed that a future pregnancy should be treated differently than my past pregnancies and that I should see a perinatologist, who specializes in high-risk pregnancies.

But that's not how my ob-gyn saw things. Despite my concerns, she saw no need to treat a subsequent pregnancy differently than she'd treated my previous pregnancies. She felt additional precautions—such as medication, testing, or increased monitoring—weren't needed. In fact, she saw no reason to involve a specialist.

In addition, when I did actually become pregnant again, she informed me that her schedule and practice location would be changing and that her time with patients would be much more limited. It was yet another indication that perhaps I was no longer in the right place.

Despite the positive doctor-patient relationship we'd had during our years together, I'd begun to see that red flag waving again, warning me that continuing a relationship with my current provider wasn't in my best interest or that of my newly conceived baby.

While she viewed my subsequent pregnancy as normal and felt comfortable treating it that way, past experience and intuition told me that no matter how healthy my pregnancy might be, it would never *truly* be normal. Not with the loss and devastation that had preceded it, and not with the unknowns and concerns surrounding those experiences.

I knew it was time to move on, but that didn't make the process any less nerve-racking. Change can be scary, even in the best of circumstances. The logical part of my brain made the decision easy, but the emotional part, not so much. It felt like a breakup, and I found myself rehearsing how I would break the news of my departure from her care. I felt as if I were betraying someone who'd been a confidante during the most difficult times in my life. I was afraid of offending her. Not to mention that we'd been together for so long, and it's never easy to sever a relationship. In truth, I felt guilty because I truly liked her as a person.

I was also concerned about all that would be lost in switching to a new provider. My ob-gyn knew me. She knew my history and heartbreak firsthand, and I was worried that the bare bones of a medical record wouldn't convey the full gravity of my circumstances. I was concerned that important information would be missed, that my new provider would dismiss my fear of another loss as well as the conviction that my pregnancy needed a higher level of supervision. But I also knew that change was necessary, and I was trusting God to lead me through the fear, uncertainty, and tricky emotions.

I researched, prayed, and practiced my breakup speech before ultimately making a decision based on the information outside of me and the intuition inside of me. With any number of providers to choose from, it was no accident that I landed on the one who would walk me through the entirety of my pregnancy, meeting each of my needs before I even expressed them to her.

From the very beginning I knew it was a relationship arranged by God. My new provider, a midwife, already had a wonderful working relationship with the specialist I'd chosen. In fact, she referred me to the specialist before realizing that I'd already begun working with her on my own. My midwife offered testing, arranged services, and gave specific options for labor and delivery before I even thought to ask for them. She met my pregnancy after loss with equal parts compassion and firmness, both of which were needed. And my very first appointment with her filled me with an indescribable sense of peace.

As with anything related to pregnancy after loss, the process of finding a new provider can be challenging and emotionally draining. It can cause anxiety. It's not a decision to be taken lightly because we know that our well-being, and that of our babies, depends at least partially on the prenatal care we receive.

Maybe you're already working with a provider you love. Maybe you have no doubt that you are receiving the best care possible. Maybe you are confident in your provider's plan. If so, I'm truly glad because your relationship with your medical provider is so important.

But if you're questioning that relationship, if your intuition doesn't match up with the guidance, or lack thereof, coming from your provider, it's okay to proceed with the it's-not-you-it's-me breakup speech and move on—guilt-free. After all, you are a mother to the precious baby you're growing, and you of all people have permission to seek and secure the best possible care for your child.

God has given us, as mothers, the gift of intuition, and we shouldn't be afraid to use it.

> Who has put wisdom in the inward parts
> or given understanding to the mind?
> (Job 38:36 ESV)

While we certainly can't claim to know everything, with the help of the Holy Spirit and prayer, our gut feelings can give us insight. We're never going to have all the answers, nor will the best doctors in the world, but when we know our circumstances call for change, we can trust God to lead us in the right direction. As mothers, we can trust our God-given intuition to help us make good decisions for the well-being of our children.

God, you know how complicated pregnancy after loss is. You know how hard it can be for me to listen to the intuition you've given me as a mother when others dismiss it or treat me as if I'm simply being overly cautious. But most of all, you know me and are aware of my needs and the needs of my baby. God, help me to be courageous enough to follow your promptings when my intuition begins waving that red flag. There are so many decisions to make regarding how to proceed on this journey, and I ask that you give me wisdom when making them, especially when it comes to medical care. I know the life of my baby is truly in your hands, but I also know that you have placed skilled medical providers on this earth to assist pregnant women like me in caring for the vulnerable lives you have placed within us. Guide me with your wisdom when it comes to seeking medical care—and especially if the time comes to make changes to my care plan. I know that all wisdom comes from you. Help me to hear you and to trust the knowledge you've given me.

REFLECTION

How has your God-given intuition presented itself during loss and pregnancy after loss? How have you responded to it?

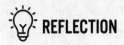

LETTER

Write a letter to your baby describing your medical journey together so far. How have your providers helped or hindered this experience?

Day 10

CHOOSING TO FOCUS ON YOUR PREGNANCY INSTEAD OF ENVYING HERS

A heart at peace gives life to the body,
but envy rots the bones.

—PROVERBS 14:30

My guess is that you've run into her everywhere you go, no matter how much you've tried to avoid the encounter. You know who I'm talking about. *Her*—the woman who is blissfully pregnant, unaware of the possibility that pregnancy could indeed break her heart.

For many weeks during the early stages of my pregnancy, my evening routine consisted of successfully avoiding *her* by settling into bed well before nightfall to lose myself in one of my favorite sitcoms.

It had become my safe place, my bubble, where I wouldn't have to answer questions about my growing belly or inadvertently come into contact with pregnant women or newborn babies.

With the wounds of loss still open, such sights resulted in emotional turmoil. The grief over what I had lost poured out while resentment seeped in, gripping my heart. In an effort to shield myself from the hurt and to stabilize my feelings, I took refuge in my bed, a place where I could control what was allowed to enter my small, isolated world.

But one evening when my cell phone rang, the bubble popped.

The caller ID indicated it was my brother. Since we aren't generally a family that calls just to say hello, I suspected he had some important news to share. A feeling of dread rose from the pit of my stomach as instinct told me there was a pregnancy announcement waiting for me on the other end of the line.

So, I didn't answer because I was afraid.

Afraid of what my response would be if my instincts were correct. Afraid I wouldn't be able to fake happiness for my brother and his wife. Afraid that my sister-in-law would get to keep her baby and I wouldn't get to keep mine. Afraid that their baby, who I later learned was due just three weeks after mine, would come to be a reminder of what I didn't have.

I decided to call my brother back. I knew that whatever news awaited wasn't going to go away.

Better to get it over with.

The conversation started out with small talk before he stated that he had some news to share. And before he could continue, I asked if he and his wife were expecting another baby. He confirmed that they were, but I could not muster a congratulatory word. It was a matter-of-fact conversation that ended with a simple acknowledgment that I'd heard what he'd said.

And with that, the fear that had been pulsing through my veins was quickly replaced with envy. Unfortunately, I was all too familiar with that soul-sucking feeling. In fact, it had been a part of me since that first time I stepped out from an exam room after discovering a baby I deeply wanted was gone. I had scanned the hospital lobby for my husband, but instead I had seen *her*—a pregnant woman with a smile as wide as the space between heaven and earth. I had felt the tears begin streaming down my cheeks as Luke approached, and he had reached me just in time for my sobs to be muffled by burying my face in his chest.

Then Micah was stillborn, and it suddenly felt as if I were surrounded by pregnant women at every turn. They were at church, school, the grocery store, the gym, the dentist's office. They were quite literally everywhere, and no matter how hard I tried, I could not prevent myself from coming into contact with them. I couldn't help but notice the babies that were being added to families all around me, while my own had been subtracted from ours.

I figured that becoming pregnant again would void these feelings of envy, but instead of going away, they simply changed.

I looked at pregnant women around me, including those close to me whom I loved, and I was consumed by a desire to have what they had. A normal pregnancy. One in which I could walk forward with confidence that my baby would become a permanent fixture in our family. One in which I wasn't concerned with the statistics and wouldn't think about how many pregnant women I knew and worry that it would be me who would lose my baby. One in which I wasn't afraid that someone else's happiness would result in my heartache.

It was a strange place to be. I was carrying a baby I had begged God for, yet those feelings of envy drained the joy right out of me. I assumed all those normal pregnancies would result in the birth of a living baby. And somehow, those positive outcomes would negatively affect mine.

Maybe you find yourself in a similar position right now, envious of the ease with which others are walking through pregnancy, desperately wishing you still had the privilege of naivete and were oblivious to the possibilities of all that could go wrong.

I hope you know those feelings are normal. Who wouldn't want to return to a life that didn't involve loss? Or go back to a world in which you didn't realize that babies die? Who wouldn't want to carry a baby in her womb, completely unaware of the heartbreak that could result from it?

I know I wanted that.

But allowing envy to take up space in my heart left little room for much else. It suffocated the joy I so badly wanted to feel in light of an answered prayer. It drew my attention toward the goodness in others' lives, causing me to stomp right past the goodness in my own. It lured me into a constant state of anxiety, believing that another woman's pregnancy had anything to do with mine.

Maybe you can relate. Maybe envy has blocked your awareness of the goodness present in your own circumstances. Your own pregnancy. Your own baby.

It's so easy to get wrapped up in the beauty of everyone else's circumstances, isn't it? To compare what they have to what we don't. To let what they have steal the joy from what we have. But in doing so, we become blind to the beauty right in front of us.

Pregnancy after loss is hard. With it comes the burden of grief and uncertainty. And while the guarantee of a living baby would surely bring peace to an anxious mama's heart, it would only be temporary. Because trouble never really ends this side of heaven; it just changes. However, that doesn't mean we cannot access peace from moment to moment.

When envy sinks into your bones, causing emotional upheaval within, cry out to God. Breathe in his peace. He has so much more for you beyond the difficulties of your current circumstances. Breathe out the envy, the emotions that tell you what you perceive to be good in *her* life somehow impacts the possibility of God doing something good in *your* life.

Envy only has the power you give it. Don't allow it to take your entire being hostage and keep you from seeing the beauty in the life you are carrying.

Friend, look down at your belly and be comforted knowing there is a much-wanted life growing within you right now. God did not choose those other women to carry your beautiful baby—he chose you. He equipped you for the task of mothering this child, regardless of what that entails. Take heart in knowing that he has not left you and will not leave you to do it alone.

God, I come to you with envy in my heart. I hate feeling this way, but I look around and see so many other babies. It makes me afraid that I won't get to keep mine. I worry that I am going to be left with empty arms again. God, I thank you for this baby that you have so graciously placed within my womb, that I have the privilege to mother for as long as you will allow. Help me to focus on what you have given me to carry instead of what others are carrying. Let me find peace in knowing that you are walking this journey of pregnancy and motherhood with me, and that no matter what happens, you will not leave me to do it alone. God, empty my heart of envy so I can make room for joy.

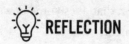

REFLECTION

Envy has been described as pain in the face of another's good fortune. How would you characterize the pain of envy as you've experienced it in connection with pregnancy? In what ways has it crowded out the joy you could be experiencing right now?

LETTER

Focusing on gratitude often helps to ease the pain of envy. Talk to your baby about how grateful you are that God chose you to be his or her mother. Be specific, listing three to five things for which you are grateful right now.

Day 11

THE COURAGE TO BELIEVE GOD
MADE YOUR BODY CAPABLE

I praise you because I am fearfully and
wonderfully made;
your works are wonderful,
I know that full well.

—PSALM 139:14

With each passing day of my pregnancy, I wondered if my body could do it—if it could carry my baby first to the stage of viability and then to a point at which the chance for life was greater than the chance for death.

My body had failed me and my babies twice before.

When referring to my losses, people often commented on how there must have been something wrong with my babies. How they surely must have had chromosomal abnormalities or a mystery illness or were otherwise unhealthy. Because when a woman loses a baby during pregnancy, people tend to assume that the baby just wasn't strong enough to survive.

But sometimes, for whatever reason and through no fault of her own, it's a woman's body that isn't strong enough for her baby to survive. Because, like everything else, our bodies are not immune to the devastating effects of this broken world.

If people had seen my medical records, they would have known that my losses had nothing to do with my babies and everything to do with my body. It was my body that had failed to properly implant the fertilized egg, my body that had deteriorated and gone into labor too soon despite the perfect health of the baby I was carrying. It was my body that had been incapable of carrying and nurturing not just one pregnancy but two. There was something wrong with my body, not my babies.

And I carried that knowledge with me into my subsequent pregnancy.

As my pregnancy after losing Micah progressed, almost anything could spin my mind into a frenzy. Panic was never more than a breath away. Every time I bent over or sneezed or carried something from one room to another, I worried the pressure and weight would cause my water to break, sending me into premature labor again.

Standing, sitting, walking, rolling over in bed—basically any type of motion whatsoever—were causes for concern. I worried that simply moving would cause me to lose my baby. And when a series of seasonal illnesses made any type of mobility nearly impossible due to aching bones and fatigue, I wondered if my body could withstand both a weakened immune system and a high-risk pregnancy.

To outsiders, these likely seem to be irrational fears. But to someone who has experienced loss, the idea that something so minor could be responsible for a major casualty feels completely rational. Especially when you have no concrete answers about why the loss occurred in the first place.

I desperately wanted to believe that my body was capable of bringing another baby safely into this world, but all I could think about were the many ways it had failed me in the past. It's hard to imagine your body producing a living being when you know so intimately its ability to destroy one.

But here's the thing: our bodies are fearfully and wonderfully made by the very capable hands of our God. In fact, the Bible tells us we are created in God's own image (Genesis 1:27) and that he himself believes our bodies to be good. These flesh-and-blood structures that house our hearts and souls and babies are proof of God's power to create us in and for his glory.

As women, we are specifically designed to be vessels of life; to carry babies within us and birth them out of our very own bodies when the time comes.

While it's true that our bodies don't always function as God intended, that's not by God's design. It's because we live in a world that doesn't always function as God intended. Everything about this world is far from perfect. It's broken and bleeding and begging for relief. Which sounds familiar, right?

But just as this world is not beyond repair by the hands of a mighty God, neither is your body. And just as we can choose to appreciate the beauty of nature despite our knowledge of its ability to cause destruction, we can choose to appreciate the beauty of our bodies even when we know they sometimes cause great disappointment.

The failure of my body had twice left my heart in shambles,

and when I became pregnant again, I sometimes felt foolish for hanging on to the hope that it might produce a different result. I struggled to believe my body was capable of doing the things God had created it to do.

But what I didn't consider was that it was already doing those things. Minute by minute, one cautious breath at a time, it was doing what it was supposed to do. It had not only conceived a precious child, but it was also carrying that precious child. And even with the knowledge that my body could be responsible for both life and death, the fact that it was carrying a baby at all was a wonderful work of God. My body was working as God intended, at least for the time being. And that was no small thing.

God chose my body to carry a very specific baby. He chose me to mother a very specific child. And while there was no telling how long I would be able to do either, the fact that I had the opportunity to do these things at all was a reason to praise the One who made me.

Now, don't get me wrong. Second by second, I begged God to let me keep this one—to allow me to carry my child outside of my womb too. I wasn't living in a bubble of ignorant bliss. I knew that at any moment, I might have to say goodbye. And just as with my two previous pregnancies, I knew that a few weeks or a few months with my baby in the womb would never be enough time. I didn't want to mother another child in heaven while I was still on earth.

But I cannot deny that my pregnancy was a sacred work of God, regardless of the outcome. Nor can I deny that my body is, and my pregnancy was, proof of God's glorious work. No one else has the power to form such a marvelous creation out of nothing.

When you are worried that your body isn't capable, remember

that God is more than capable. Cling to the hope that in carrying this baby, your body is already doing what it's supposed to do. And day by day, as your body expands with the growth of your child, trust that God has your best interests at heart. He created your body for his purposes, and he will see that those purposes are carried out.

Your body may have disappointed you in the most heart-breaking of ways. It might, in fact, be broken. But some of God's best work takes place in brokenness. And while there are no promises when it comes to pregnancy, you can be assured that God will use your body for his glory, in one way or another. For you are one of his greatest works, and your life in this body is not to be wasted.

God, I praise you for creating my body and the body of my unborn child in your perfect image. My body and the one I'm carrying within are nothing short of miracles, proof of your glorious works. I worry that my body will fail again, that it won't be able to nurture the vulnerable life of my baby, that it will not be able to carry out the functions for which you designed it. I so desperately want the opportunity to raise the child you have placed within me, to watch him or her grow outside of my body. But I fear my body is too broken to carry my baby through a successful pregnancy. God, remind me that you are capable even when I'm not and that your purposes for my body are higher than my own. Remind me that you have created my body with intention and that nothing you create goes to waste. You are a God whose works are wonderful, and that does not change even when life doesn't feel that way. Help me to embrace peace in knowing that you are capable of all things.

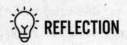

REFLECTION

Take a good look at your body and write down at least three things about it for which you are grateful. In what ways is God's glory already evident in and through your body?

LETTER

Describe to your baby the ways your body has blessed you during your pregnancy so far.

Day 12

THE COURAGE TO SEEK COMFORT
IN GOD INSTEAD OF GOOGLE

*"Come to me, all you who are weary and
burdened, and I will give you rest."*
—MATTHEW 11:28

Promise me one thing," said my perinatologist during our first appointment together after I became pregnant with my son. "Promise me that you'll stay off Google."

She was totally serious. She promised to provide the best possible care for me and my unborn baby, and because she knew that keeping me from getting lost in the vastness of the internet would truly be in my best interest, she asked for just that one small promise in return.

With her years of experience working with women who were enduring high-risk and mentally taxing pregnancies, she knew that patients like me ached for answers, for guarantees, for peace. And she knew that with the ability to google every symptom, every concern, every possible outcome of pregnancy, patients like me had a tendency to rely on Google to provide those things, to seek out comfort in internet answers when it inevitably provided anything but.

She didn't want my already tangled mind to get caught in the speculations and worst-case scenarios of the World Wide Web. Where one heartbreaking story leads to a hundred more. Where it's too easy to convince myself that someone else's misfortune will certainly become mine. Where I absorb every horrific story of pregnancy gone wrong, of soul-crushing loss. I was carrying enough pregnancy trauma of my own—I certainly didn't need to be carrying everyone else's. My anxiety was already off the charts.

And she knew that.

So I would have been wise to make that promise and stick to it.

But instead, I smiled, nodded, and offered a weak, "Okay," knowing full well that Google would be my go-to for reassurance and advice during a difficult pregnancy. I might as well have had my fingers crossed behind my back because it was a promise I had no intention of keeping. Just as it had been after my ectopic pregnancy, then after my stillbirth, Google would be my guide. My sanctuary. My friend. My support. Google would tell me what I wanted to hear.

With each stroke of the keyboard, Google would be the keeper of my deepest fears and heartache. I was regularly feeding it information, and it was keeping track of it all, fueling an intimate relationship between the two of us.

Missed period. Baby's heartbeat. No heartbeat. Preterm labor. Pregnancy loss. Recurring loss. Statistics for successful pregnancy after loss. Pregnancy after PPROM. Thinning cervix. Amniotic sludge. Viability.

I handed over all my secrets, all my concerns. I divulged my past and present, my history and fear of the future. But the only thing I got in return was more fear, more anxiety. Each search result felt like a mockery of my greatest vulnerabilities, like a finger pointed at me, declaring how foolish I was to think that after two losses, I might have a successful pregnancy. Not one search result provided a definite answer. Not one specifically addressed my endless list of what-ifs. Not one promised that everything would be okay. Not one gave me the one thing I was truly looking for—certainty.

With such a vast amount of information available at our fingertips, it's easy to think that our hearts can be settled by something we read online. Certainly, the answers we want are out there if we can just dig deep enough into the hole of the internet to find them, right? We travel into the abyss, each link taking us further down, yet assurance escapes us. It can't be found. Not from Google, anyway.

During my pregnancy, there was no shortage of concerns to try and make sense of through the use of Google. There was my very first OB appointment in which we couldn't hear the heartbeat. There was the cervix scare. There was bed rest. There was amniotic sludge. There was conflicting information from my providers. And later on, there was a concern over a possible heart defect (which was monitored until eventually resolving itself).

I googled most of those things obsessively, searching for articles I had not yet uncovered, for answers I had not yet found. I was constantly seeking that one piece of information that would give me peace by way of certainty that my baby would be born healthy and alive.

But that never happened.

Instead of peace, I mostly felt panic as I clicked and typed and scrolled. Because it turns out, Google couldn't give me the comfort I needed, no matter how much I searched. In fact, the only time I did feel peace, at least temporarily, was when I tuned out the whirling noise inside my head and turned off the noise of my internet browser. It was then that I could still my mind and pray, truly seeking God while remembering the goodness he had lavished on me, even when I couldn't see or feel it. It was then that I was reminded of the hard places he'd already led me through and could at last focus on what I knew to be true: I was still carrying my baby and God was still carrying me.

Now, the internet isn't all bad when it comes to pregnancy after loss. Sometimes it's a healthy source of information and can provide useful facts. And I haven't forgotten the few select support groups and nonprofit organizations that were an ongoing source of hope and solidarity. There's nothing like connecting with others who truly feel your pain and understand the depth of your concerns during pregnancy after loss in a community where the lingering grief and ongoing angst are validated. Where you are surrounded by other people who share similarly difficult circumstances. That's all good and healthy.

But obsessively searching for answers online to all of our what-ifs? Reading every heartbreaking story of loss or pregnancy after loss? It will never give us what we need. Because the answers to most, if not all, of our most pressing questions don't exist this side of heaven. When googling only leaves you paralyzed with fear, it's time to seek God instead.

When we enter the presence of God, truth is revealed. And the truth is that our safety is found in God alone.

He will cover you with his feathers,
     and under his wings you will find refuge;
     his faithfulness will be your shield and
          rampart. (Psalm 91:4)

Google is unreliable. God is not. Google tends to amplify all the hard things we already have too much of: fear, anxiety, hopelessness, unrest. God is a refuge from those things. Google is heavy on speculation and light on truth. God *is* truth.

Look, I know you're not going to promise to stop googling all the things about this much-anticipated but most uncertain pregnancy. I wouldn't ask you to. But I want you to remember this: Google in moderation, God in excess. Before you get tangled up in the sticky World Wide Web, go to God. He's listening. In fact, he invites us to come to him when burdens overwhelm us and our hearts are weary. No, he may not reveal to you all of the answers you seek, but he is the only one who actually knows those answers.

No matter how many times you type "chances of baby surviving after loss" into your search bar, you're not going to get a good answer because Google doesn't know you (although the argument can be made that it just might if, like me, you've noticed that it seems to be uncomfortably familiar with your life). But you can be certain you are known and loved by a good God. Take your hurt to him. Hand your fear to him. He promises peace and rest. He's got all the answers—and even if they aren't the ones you're hoping for, you can be sure that, in time, he will reveal all you could ever want to know. But until then, you can trust him to hold your weary heart, to speak only truth, and to provide rest.

*God, I am desperate for answers to all my whys and what-ifs.
I'm desperate for certainty that my pregnancy will have the outcome I desire. I'm in such a hard place, and I've been seeking
instant comfort through information available at my fingertips.
Not surprisingly, it has failed to satisfy my unquenchable mind.
Today, I don't know how this chapter of my story will end. I
don't know the number of my baby's days. But I do know I'm
still carrying my baby and that my baby is deeply loved. In this
moment, help me to find peace in the knowledge that you have
the answers I so desperately seek. That you have a plan for my
life and the life of my baby. Help me to find the comfort I seek
in you rather than the internet. God, remind me that Google
doesn't fix the problems of this life—you do.*

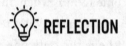

REFLECTION

*How has your internet usage impacted your emotions, for bet-
ter and for worse? In what ways, if any, are you tempted to seek
out comfort from the internet rather than from God?*

LETTER

*Let's do something different today. Instead of writing a letter to
your baby, write one to God. Lay out all of your questions, all of
the unknowns, all of your fears. Ask God to be your refuge, to
comfort you and shield you even in the midst of all these things.*

Day 13

CHANGING THE NARRATIVE ON WHAT-IF

[God] is able to do immeasurably more than all we ask or imagine, according to his power that is at work within us.
—EPHESIANS 3:20

Every trip to the bathroom was enough to push me to the brink of a nervous breakdown. I was terrified that I would find blood, often the first sign of a worst-case scenario when it comes to pregnancy. As silly as it sounds, I genuinely hated using the bathroom because I was afraid I'd come face-to-face with the harsh reality that my pregnancy was in trouble. The mere thought that I might find blood could spiral my thoughts into a million more what-ifs.

What if there's blood? became *What if I lose this baby?* and then *What if I can't get ahold of my doctor? What if I have to go to the hospital? What if my husband doesn't answer his phone? What if I never get to have another baby?*

And those were just the beginning of the what-ifs.

They followed me throughout my entire pregnancy, terrorizing me with endlessly dark possibilities of what awful things could happen.

Before every ultrasound appointment: *What if there is no heartbeat?*

After every OB appointment: *What if they missed something?*

When potential complications arose: *What if this doesn't resolve itself as expected?*

Between appointments: *What if my baby doesn't make it to the next one?*

Before I left the house to go anywhere: *What if I start bleeding?*

When I was out in public: *What if I go into premature labor?*

Before falling asleep: *What if I accidentally roll onto my back and cut off my baby's blood supply?*

When my baby wasn't moving: *What if something is wrong?*

When he seemed to be moving too much: *What if he's in distress?*

Before every church service: *What if someone mentions my pregnancy and I descend into a pool of tears?*

During labor: *What if I have another stillbirth?*

You see where I'm going with this, right? I was so focused on what could go wrong that I forfeited the joy of allowing myself to consider what might actually go right.

I rarely, if ever, pictured bringing home my son. It was too scary to imagine it only to potentially be hit with the reality of his death. So, I spent much of my pregnancy in full denial that I was carrying a baby who could actually live. As a result, there were many things I didn't do because I was afraid my what-ifs would become I-knew-its.

I didn't send formal pregnancy announcements as I had in the past. In fact, I told almost no one. When my pregnancy became obvious to those at church, my daughter's school, or other social circles, I rarely allowed for conversation about it. The waters were too murky, and I didn't want to draw attention to what was growing beneath the surface until it became clear that a life would fully emerge.

I didn't take or share photos to social media as my pregnancy progressed—another stark contrast to what I'd done in the past. It felt too vulnerable. Too foolish. It would have invited too many questions, too many false hopes, and too much exposure in the event one of those what-ifs became a reality.

I didn't have a baby shower or decorate a nursery. How could I have feigned the joy that is expected from women who are pregnant when my reality held so much lament? And what if I ended up with a roomful of baby clothes, accessories, necessities, and decor, but ultimately didn't have a baby who would use all those things?

I didn't talk in terms of when my baby would arrive but *if* he did—*if* he came home. Because what if he didn't?

For mamas like us, the list of what-ifs during pregnancy is endless. But I suspect you already know that. For as many as I've discussed here, you know there are so many more. And you know they can truly make you feel trapped in a cycle of hopelessness.

My what-ifs held me captive. They bound me in a perpetual state of discouragement as I allowed my mind to pace incessantly in the confines of worry. Instead of focusing on God's infinite capabilities, I focused on my own perceived incapabilities and lack of control. Instead of taking my thoughts captive and resting in the knowledge that there is always hope with God, I let the what-ifs steal my joy.

And I regret that.

> We take captive every thought to make it obedient to Christ.
> (2 Corinthians 10:5)

I regret that, during what turned out to be my last pregnancy, I was distracted from the miracle of it all—from the gift that is pregnancy. From the opportunity to carry my baby with a sense of joy instead of intense fear. Never again will I carry a baby in my womb, and I wish I'd allowed myself to enjoy my final pregnancy even just a smidgen more. And yet, I know it's easier said than done.

I thought that by preparing myself for the worst, I was somehow protecting myself. That if I lost another baby, it would somehow be less devastating if I actually planned for it. And, well, if my baby lived, what a grand surprise that would be!

But I was fooling myself. Expecting my baby to die wouldn't shelter me from the excruciating pain and grief if the worst did happen.

Author Brené Brown addresses this type of thinking in her book *Daring Greatly.*

> We can't prepare for tragedy and loss. When we turn every opportunity to feel joy into a test drive for despair, we actually diminish our resilience. Yes, softening into joy is uncomfortable. Yes, it's scary. Yes, it's vulnerable. *But every time we allow ourselves to lean into joy and give in to those moments, we build resilience and we cultivate hope.* The joy becomes part

of who we are, and when bad things happen—and they do happen—we are stronger.[1]

Did you catch that part about leaning into joy and cultivating hope? Allowing ourselves to feel joy promotes hope, and hope is a necessary ingredient in the mixture of emotions during pregnancy after loss.

To be clear, your concerns are no doubt valid, as are your feelings—yes, even the negative ones. The what-ifs are an unavoidable factor in pregnancy after loss. But here are a few more what-ifs to consider: What if your what-ifs didn't have to control you like they did me? What if you could change the narrative of your what-ifs, or at least add a dose of optimism to them? What if you could soften into joy?

I'm not suggesting that you completely cut the what-ifs from your pregnancy experience. Nor would I expect you to. But I do want to challenge you to respond to them differently.

When you think, *What if the worst happens?* choose to respond with, *What if it doesn't?*

What if your baby doesn't die?

What if your just-born baby lets out the sharp cry you so desperately long to hear?

What if you leave the hospital with your arms full?

What if you bring your precious baby home?

I know you're afraid. So was I. But when you get caught in the self-defeating spiral of those what-ifs, don't forget that we worship a God who has the power to do so much more than we can fathom. He is all-powerful and beyond capable of delivering that sweet baby right into your arms, alive and well.

What if he doesn't, you ask?

To that I respond: What if he does? What if God reveals his power through your pregnancy? What if he already has? What if, as you hold your newborn baby snug against your chest, God's glory looks you right in the face through the sleepy eyes of your precious child?

Go ahead and ask yourself those hard what-ifs. But remember to also ask the what-ifs that fill you with hope.

God, the what-ifs surrounding my pregnancy are too numerous to count. My fears are real and overwhelming. Because so many of them have been realized in the past, I know it's possible for them to again become a reality. My mind so easily spirals into a place of defeat as the what-ifs pile up, crushing my hope. But I'm tired of being held captive by them and of the hopelessness they produce. Help me to escape this captivity by asking "what if" in another light—the light that reminds me you are capable of far more than I can comprehend. Please restore joy to my pregnancy by helping me to focus on your goodness instead of the grief of this world. I don't know how the what-ifs will play out, but I trust that your glory will shine whether this pregnancy ends in darkness or light.

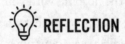 **REFLECTION**

Write down three fearful what-ifs. For each one, write out a corresponding hopeful what-if. Elaborate on the hopeful what-ifs by describing what you imagine the outcomes might be if the best-case scenario happens.

LETTER

Set aside the worst-case what-ifs and write a letter to your baby addressing the best-case what-ifs. For example, what if you bring your baby home? What do you imagine that will look like? How will you feel?

Day 14

THE COURAGE TO ASK FOR AND ACCEPT HELP

We must help the weak, remembering the words the Lord Jesus himself said: "It is more blessed to give than to receive."
—ACTS 20:35

I paged through a magazine on the couch, feigning a calm I did not feel. In fact, I was incredibly uncomfortable.

The discomfort wasn't related to my rapidly expanding waistline. It had nothing to do with the weight of a tiny, growing human that pressed against my organs, nor was it related to my sore back and never-quite-settled stomach.

No, the cause of my discomfort was embarrassment, even shame, from watching my mother-in-law complete housework in *my* house. Chores that I, a grown woman, should have been capable of doing myself.

The sight of the perfectly straight lines she carved into the carpet with my vacuum made me wince. I felt somewhat disgusted with myself for having this woman do my dirty work—*and* do it better than me under normal circumstances. Not only that, but she had traveled many hours by car to do so. Guilt weaseled its way into my consciousness because I was certain she'd never enlisted the help of anyone else, especially her mother-in-law, to vacuum her floors while she kicked up her feet.

My husband and I had asked for her help, as well as that of my father-in-law, and they had agreed to do so without complaint. But I wouldn't say it felt good.

Similar scenarios resurfaced again and again as I transferred the baton of everyday tasks to the hands of others during the course of what felt like the longest pregnancy ever recorded.

Questions remained about how much work was safe for me to do during my pregnancy. Though I was on strict bed rest for just a short time, the conflicting opinions and advice of my medical team that came afterward blurred the line between overly cautious and too risky. While one provider encouraged me to stay off my feet and enlist as much help as possible, the other believed it was safe to engage in normal activities.

But I could not escape the words "do as little as possible—just to be safe" from my midwife, regardless of how well my pregnancy seemed to be progressing or how optimistic my specialist was. So I erred on the side of overly cautious. I reasoned I could either recruit a small village to help me bring my baby home or I could stand alone, determined to do it myself at the (potential) expense of my baby—and my heart.

The way I saw it, those were my only two options.

Had I spent those long months heaving the vacuum up and down the stairs, hauling in groceries, scrubbing floors, being the sole caregiver for my daughter, and completing every other day-to-day task without any help at all, my pregnancy may very well have still progressed normally. But I wasn't willing to take that chance. So, when others asked how they could help, I told them. And when they didn't ask, I still told them.

I'll never forget the drive home from my specialist's office immediately after the cervix scare early on in my pregnancy. I was shaken, believing I had narrowly averted a crisis. Even so, I wanted to tell my mom that all was well for the time being. When I explained the doctor's concerns and my own, she immediately offered to help.

She traveled several hours every other week during months with some of the harshest weather to tend to me, her fully grown and should-be-capable daughter. And while the guilt I felt for enlisting the help of my own mother wasn't as heavy as it was for accepting help from my mother-in-law, it still loomed. Because while she's a hardy and energetic woman, I had no doubt that the ongoing back-and-forth travel and physical labor of housekeeping and childcare were taking a toll. Not only had she already served her time in such roles, but she still had her own work and responsibilities to tend to.

Friends offered up countless meals. Even when the demands of work schedules and managing their own busy households kept them from doing anything else, they could fill our plates alongside their own.

Numerous times I requested help with childcare, sometimes paid, sometimes unpaid, at least partially because I wanted my daughter to have the undivided attention I found difficult to give her as I wrestled with the combination of grief and fear that colored my days.

I also asked far more of my husband than I can imagine

relationship experts would deem fair. The division of labor within our home was far from equal. And yet, I continued to ask because my broken spirit needed the help. Every day, my husband wearied himself with his full-time job before coming home to take care of the household and child-rearing duties I hadn't managed to complete. His spirit was depleted, too, yet he carried on without complaint knowing that my well-being was essential for the well-being of our baby.

Looking back, I'm not surprised that I battled feelings of unworthiness and failure. As a stay-at-home mom, I felt I was surely starting to resemble that old (and completely inaccurate) stereotype of the woman who spends her day watching her favorite soap operas while eating bonbons. Had anyone asked me during those months, "So, what do you do all day?" I wouldn't have had an answer.

I needed help to keep my body from becoming physically overworked and my psyche from becoming mentally overloaded. Because, as you probably know, pregnancy after loss requires an inordinate amount of mental labor when every day consists of concurrently willing yourself to believe your baby is going to make it while also preparing for the worst-case scenario. Again.

Now, don't get me wrong—I greatly appreciated the help. And sure, it was nice to have other people take over some of the less-than-thrilling responsibilities of everyday life. I was grateful that our small circle was enough to surround us with the support we needed. But it never feels good to be the one who always seems to be reaching out for help when everyone else seems to be functioning normally.

I can't know what your exact situation entails. Maybe you work full-time, or maybe you're an around-the-clock caretaker. Maybe your work is done at a desk, or perhaps it requires more physical exertion. Maybe you're on bed rest, or maybe you're maintaining your normal exercise routine. Maybe you're experiencing pregnancy complications, or maybe things are progressing normally.

What I do know is this: being pregnant after losing a baby is an incredibly difficult season. And even if we can easily acknowledge this reality, asking for and accepting help is still hard. We don't always like the idea of receiving help because it can make us feel like a burden, which might be a consequence of living in a culture that never stops telling us we should be able to overcome any hardship we face on our own.

But that's not what God says. Scripture makes it clear that we are not expected to do this life alone. After all, we are told to seek God's help and to help one another. And when we are the ones who happen to need help? Well, there's no shame in that.

> Share with the Lord's people who are in need. Practice hospitality. (Romans 12:13)

There are seasons in which we are the helpers and doers, in which we are strong and capable. And then there are seasons in which we are the recipients of help, when weakness proves our human limits, when we need to be strengthened by God and held up by those around us.

Pregnancy after loss is one such season.

Friend, you may be the only one carrying your baby, but you don't have to carry the entire load of this pregnancy by yourself. Yes, it is an amazing gift, but we know that doesn't mean it's easy.

It's okay to ask for help without clothing yourself in layers of guilt. It's okay to accept help without feeling indebted to those who offer it. Because the people who can help you in this season? Well, they want what's best for you and your baby too. And while they don't have the power to change your circumstances, they can help you through them. They can support the well-being of your unborn baby. Is there a better gift to give or receive than one that might be instrumental in bringing a new and precious life into this world?

I sure can't think of one.

It can be uncomfortable to ask for help, and it can be uncomfortable to accept help. It takes courage and vulnerability to say, "Right now, I am weak," and admit that outside help might be just what you need.

But we are told to help the weak—and right now, that might mean you. That's okay. I pray that others will take the initiative to offer up help, but if not, don't be afraid to ask. You weren't created to do everything by yourself, and when you admit your weaknesses, God provides a way.

God, most days I wonder how I am going to do this. I am one person who is literally carrying the weight of another human life, and after losing a baby, I feel unequipped to bring life into this world again. As grateful as I am for this pregnancy, I cannot deny that it is draining and difficult on so many levels. I could sure use some help, but I feel embarrassed to ask. I feel ashamed when other people do the work I think I should be doing myself. I feel guilty for burdening others with the difficult circumstances of my life. And sometimes, I wonder if there is even anyone to help me. But you make it clear, God, that we are human and therefore carry with us intrinsic weaknesses. I understand that we are not made to endure the trials of this life alone. When I need help, help me to be vulnerable enough to ask for it. And when I receive an offer of help, give me the ability to accept it with a heart of gratitude instead of a heart of guilt. Help me to truly believe that accessing the strength of those around me is in the best interest of my baby, and there's no shame in that.

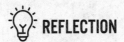

REFLECTION

What needs, if any, are you reluctant to ask for or to accept help with? What thoughts or emotions arise when you consider asking for the help you need? If you are willing, choose one need and identify one or two people you will ask to help you with that need.

LETTER

Tell your baby about the people in your life who have supported you on this journey of pregnancy after loss. What have they done for you, and what do they mean to you?

Day 15

HOLDING FAST TO THE ASSURANCE OF WHAT CANNOT BE TAKEN FROM YOU

*"I have told you these things, so that in me you may
have peace. In this world you will have trouble.
But take heart! I have overcome the world."*

—JOHN 16:33

Do you know what people sometimes forget? They forget that I'm not just a woman who has lost babies but a woman who remains a mother to those babies. It's almost as if there's an assumption that when my babies were stripped from this world, so was my title as their mother.

But just as my babies became part of me when they came to life in my body, so did my title as their mother. And even though they didn't remain, I did—and I carry their memory with me.

Yes, I lost Micah and the unnamed baby of my ectopic pregnancy. But I still claim them as my children. I carried them. My body was their home. While they grew within me, my heart grew too. I loved them then and I love them now. And even though they are in heaven, one day I'll be with them there too.

It took some time for me to realize all this. That even though my babies had been taken, my position as their mother hadn't. It wasn't the motherhood experience I would ever have asked for. Never would I have wanted to experience so much sorrow and heartbreak, but these things are nevertheless a considerable part of my motherhood story.

While I wouldn't suggest that this realization made loss easier, it did create a sense of comfort. No one can remove my title as mother to the babies who didn't come home with me. No one can tell me I'm not their mother. No one can take away the memories of positive pregnancy tests or ultrasounds showing a mysteriously exquisite creature bouncing off the walls of my uterus. No one can take away the memory of a heartbeat filling the void of a sterile examination room. No one can take away the truth of their existence that's etched into my entire being. No one can take away my love for them. And even in the face of the hopelessness of loss, no one can take away my hope in knowing that this story isn't over.

Do you know what else can't be taken away? God's love for my babies—and for me. Even in the midst of the ugliness of grief. Even in the uncertainty. Even in the deeply rooted anxiety of pregnancy after loss that was planted when two of my babies left the womb before having a chance to live.

All of this is part of what makes a subsequent pregnancy so hard. It's complicated because even though it's incredibly beautiful, we know that beautiful things still wither and die. We wonder if the soil is fertile enough to nourish a pregnancy into a breathing life. But even with the knowledge that it might not be, even with the anxiety and fear that extend so deeply into the experience of pregnancy after loss, there's something else that can't be taken. And that's hope.

Hope still grows. And with a new life inside of you, or at least the possibility of a new life inside you, how can it not? The presence of new life—the idea of it—has a way of cultivating hope, despite the difficult circumstances surrounding it.

During my subsequent pregnancy, time and time again I cried out to God in distress. *Are you going to take this baby from me too? How will I survive another loss?*

And somewhere deep inside, a whisper reverberated the same message over and over. *In the same way you've survived the other two.*

In other words, I would survive another loss with the help of God. With the hope of heaven. With the promise that the sorrows of this earth aren't forever. And with the clasping of hands with other women who understood the devastation of loss and the delicate existence of pregnancy after loss that I hoped would help restore my heart.

Friend, I know you are clinging so tightly to this baby, that prayers for this child's well-being and survival are in constant rotation. I know that you are considering all the possibilities. That you are wondering how you'll survive another worst-case scenario. I know these things because I've walked the road you're trudging right now, my feet beaten and blistered too.

There is a chance that this baby, your deeply longed-for baby, might be taken from you before you're ready to let go. And while I hate even thinking such things, I want to come alongside you in the hard truth that sometimes babies die, and I know how terrifying that possibility is. I want to acknowledge that the despair wrapped up in this reality is very real.

At the same time, I also want to nourish the seeds of hope in you.

Did you know that 85 percent of pregnancies that occur after one loss, and 75 percent of pregnancies that occur after two or three losses, are successful, resulting in a dewy-skinned, wiggling baby?[2] It's true! And while I validate and empathize with your likely and understandable response of, "Yes, but there's still a 15 to 25 percent chance that it won't happen," I want to gently ask you to consider that just maybe you won't fall into the latter statistic.

It doesn't make sense—loss and the complexity of life after loss. It doesn't make sense that any of us have been asked to endure such trials. But you know what else doesn't make sense? The existence of the baby you're carrying right now. The reality that in all its darkness, death has created space for life, even when it's not the reality you would have chosen. And let's not forget your courageous ability to risk loving a baby again after you've lost one.

We don't get to know ahead of time how our pregnancies will turn out. We don't get to know just exactly how our motherhood stories will unfold. There are no certainties.

I can't give you a special recipe that will guarantee you a healthy pregnancy and living baby. But perhaps I can offer a few ideas to help you create and savor hope. Perhaps I can encourage you to grasp these fleeting moments of pregnancy, no matter how difficult it might be, and carve them into your memory. Because regardless of what happens, these moments of your precious pregnancy cannot be taken from you. Nor can the value of your baby's life.

Breathe in your baby's existence. Concentrate on the love

you feel for your child right now. Store the sight of that positive pregnancy test in a compartment that is forever bolted to your mind. Bottle up the sound of that precious heartbeat and catalog the ultrasound images in your memory for easy retrieval. Count kicks and relish in the movement that is so gloriously produced within you. Let your hand gently graze your belly, as it's naturally inclined to do, and take in the majesty of this moment in which you are carrying your baby.

These moments will inevitably come to an end because this season of life is just that—a season. But they can't be taken from you.

It's in moments such as these that I wish for you to feel the presence of God and let that presence carry you forward. With the knowledge of all that can go wrong, it's so easy to surrender hope to our circumstances. But we don't have to let uncertainty about the future steal our hope.

The worry that has your insides in knots when you consider the possibility of this precious life being taken from you is real and valid and more than understandable. But I want to gently remind you that even in the midst of difficult circumstances, harsh realities, and ongoing uncertainty, we can find peace and assurance in things that cannot be taken away.

In addition to your motherhood and the endless love that goes along with it, you have this precious time with your baby. Right now. But more than that, you are promised redemption from even the most heartbreaking of circumstances. You have heaven, where your broken heart will be restored and you will join the babies to whom you've said goodbye. You have the love of a good God. And you have hope for a future in which loss no longer has the power to control your life.

Our trials, our broken hearts, our anxieties about the future of our children's lives—these things tend to hold a certain power over us. But let's remember that God holds the power over our circumstances. And even when those are awful, he is good; even when they change, he does not.

God, I'm so afraid that my baby—another one—is going to be taken away; that you're not going to allow me to keep this one either. The possibility of another loss, another devastating jab at my motherhood, makes my heart race and my mind spin. I'm afraid this pregnancy and my chance to mother this child on earth are going to be cut short, and so my fear stifles my hope. Even though I know our futures are secure in heaven, it doesn't make this experience any easier. You have made me this child's mother, and while the circumstances aren't what I would have chosen, help me cling to the truth that I will always hold that position. These beautiful moments of motherhood right now cannot be taken from me, and even with fear swirling around me, I am grateful. Thank you for your promise that the trials of this earth are temporary and that something better awaits not just for me but also for my baby. Thank you for choosing me to be this child's mother.

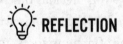 **REFLECTION**

Consider some of the most memorable and beautiful moments of your pregnancy thus far. Knowing that these can never be taken from you, how might you use these moments to help your hope grow?

LETTER

Describe some of these memorable and beautiful moments to your baby. Share what it means to you to know you will always be this child's mother, no matter what.

Day 16

THE COURAGE TO LET GRIEF AND JOY DANCE

Jesus wept.

—JOHN 11:35

It was the beginning of another week of (thankfully) being pregnant when my face contorted into blubbering sobs upon meeting with Annabel's teacher. Over the weekend, my husband and I had informed our little girl that her brother was growing inside my belly. I can only imagine that the news fired from her mouth like a cannonball as soon as she entered the classroom that day. Or maybe it was just that the billowy tops and oversized sweaters I'd been wearing weren't veiling my pregnancy as well as I'd thought.

"Congratulations!" the teacher offered when I arrived to collect my child, after the other parents had ushered their children away.

There was just something about another person's unadulterated and naive joy about my pregnancy that was hard to swallow.

And as was apt to happen when that word was directed at me, the tears burst forth, followed by an only slightly coherent explanation for why. I'm not even sure I said thank you before launching into an exposition on the reality of the situation—my losses, my grief, and my fear that the pregnancy would result in more of the same.

"I'm sorry," I sputtered, apologizing for crying. "I'm just scared," I said, feeling grateful that there were no other witnesses to my public display of affliction.

That precious teacher then hugged me and assured me she would be praying for me before sending me off, my little girl's hand in mine as, with my other hand, I continued to wipe my wet cheeks dry.

Despite feeling embarrassed by the tears over which I so obviously had no control, I felt relieved that the truth was out there. Not just about the existence of my pregnancy but about the existence of the hard and conflicting emotions that were growing along with it.

It often seemed that people overlooked the reality that my pregnancy came into existence because of loss. No one did this intentionally—Annabel's teacher hadn't known about my history of loss when she congratulated me—but it felt cruel nonetheless. And even those who did know about my history of loss weren't often inclined to acknowledge it or its effect on my subsequent pregnancy. How could they not understand I was carrying this baby only because I'd had to let another go?

I think the sorrowful tears of a pregnant woman can make people uncomfortable because sorrow and pregnancy are such a contradiction. In general, we don't imagine the two coinciding. One is associated with loss and the other with life. But what so often goes unrecognized is that pregnancy after loss is associated with both. Loss and life—or at least the possibility of life outside the womb. After loss, there is always pain attached to pregnancy. At any given point during pregnancy after loss, triggers can arise—and they *will* arise.

At twenty weeks and three days pregnant with Micah, I delivered his dead body. And do you know what I was doing at the same exact point in my subsequent pregnancy? I was gathering mementos of Micah's brief life and arranging them in a pretty box while wondering if one day I'd be doing the same thing for the baby I was carrying. I was telling my daughter about another baby I knew there was a chance she might not meet. I was trying to answer complicated questions from a little girl about her sibling in heaven and the one in my womb. And I was crying real tears from the complexity of it all after her teacher congratulated me that day.

Being pregnant after loss is a constant reminder of death, which sounds dark, doesn't it? Yes, we can tell ourselves that *this is a different pregnancy, a different baby,* which is a truth that can be a great source of hope. But we still can't separate the two—pregnancy and death. For us, death came from pregnancy, and another pregnancy came from death. The two are intertwined, no matter how glad we are to be holding a positive pregnancy test in our hands or how well our subsequent pregnancy is progressing.

I was just over halfway through what I prayed would be a full-term pregnancy when I drove Annabel home from school on that emotionally charged day. And while I did truly feel relieved by exposing some hard truths surrounding my pregnancy, I still felt embarrassed by my bumbling attempt to communicate what was actually going on behind my baby bump.

Later that evening, as had become routine during what seemed like an incredibly long and cold winter, Luke and I sat near the fireplace as Annabel danced to the music blasting from my phone. Ridiculous as it sounds, she was wearing a chicken mask, which she often did, apparently to liven up her performance.

It was silly and absurd and pure joy. And as we had so many times, and would so many more, we laughed hysterically at the ridiculousness of it all. Because it was cute and funny and precious in the way only a little girl could make such a performance.

The scene was a stark contrast from the one that had played out that morning. And looking back on all the emotions that filtered through the entirety of that day, I can't help but consider how we aren't embarrassed by such demonstrations of joy or laughter. My daughter wasn't embarrassed by her silliness and contagious giggling. My husband and I weren't embarrassed by the joy beaming from our eyes or amusement pouring from our lips.

We don't feel guilty or embarrassed for such things, nor do we feel the need to apologize for them. I suppose because they feel good and are more socially acceptable than grief and tears, which are just so uncomfortable and awkward. The slew of emotions that we'd rather not feel related to pregnancy after loss can sink us into a hole of shame and humiliation.

Which is probably where the Enemy wants us: ashamed of the emotions that accompany suffering and humiliated by the response to them. Especially when we've been granted the gift of pregnancy, when a new baby is on the horizon and we're expected to be overwhelmed with joy and gratitude, making us feel foolish when we feel anything else.

And yet we know that Jesus wept even when he knew a great miracle was about to take place, as he was the one who would perform it. Despite the fact that Jesus was about to resurrect a man named Lazarus, he wept over the man's death and joined in the heartache of those who loved him. Jesus knew the goodness that was coming, yet he still felt sorrow, and there's no indication in Scripture that he felt ashamed by it.

Similarly, you don't have to feel ashamed or embarrassed by your tears and grief. The circumstances surrounding a pregnancy that's associated with loss can hurt, and you are allowed to weep as you wait for your miracle, even when in the midst of a joyful situation. Yes, pregnancy is life and joy, hope and goodness. But pregnancy after loss is so much more. It's sorrow and death, fear and uncertainty dancing alongside the joy and anticipation of meeting the little life inside you.

And that's what this is, isn't it? A delicate dance of not just laughter and joy but grief and tears too, swaying back and forth minute by minute. Some might expect that because you are pregnant again, your grief should take a back seat to your joy. And some days it will—some days the sound of a heartbeat or impact of a little kick will sweep you off your feet. But that's not always the reality when loss has guided your steps for so long. When you're carrying a baby after losing one, it will often be grief that takes the lead, the tears from what was and what might not be *weeping* you off your feet. And some days the two will be perfectly in step. Balanced. Tears in the morning and laughter at night.

In a world that avoids the hard emotions, that sometimes even mocks them—a world that ignores the pain associated with pregnancy after loss—you don't have to hide your raw emotions, nor do you need to feel embarrassed by them. Even on the days you feel misunderstood or unseen, rest assured that God is close to your hurting heart and crushed spirit and that he's weeping over the same things you are. What others don't understand about your pregnancy, God does.

> The LORD is close to the brokenhearted
> and saves those who are crushed in spirit.
> (Psalm 34:18)

You might feel pressure to allow only joy to be your partner through this grueling dance, but when you know that even God accepts and feels sorrow at the realities of this troublesome world, you, too, can courageously embrace the presence of grief.

God, sometimes I feel embarrassed by my tears. I feel pressure to move on from the pain of loss even though I know pain is a part of this life here on earth. After all, you said it would be. But even when those around me are compassionate and empathetic, I still feel pressure to get over my grief and pull myself together. I wish that sorrow weren't part of my pregnancy; I wish my pregnancy could shine with pure joy instead of being tarnished with grief. But you remind me that you're no stranger to tears and mourning, and I thank you for showing me examples of this. Help me to honor both the joy and grief of this pregnancy and remind me that both are accepted by you, even if others dismiss my grief. Thank you for promising to be near when my heart is broken and my spirit is crushed.

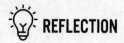 **REFLECTION**

Jesus honored his grief when he openly wept at the death of his friend Lazarus. What do you think it might mean for you to honor and embrace your grief? Consider any parallels there might be by reflecting on how you honor and embrace your joy.

 LETTER

Describe for your baby some of your greatest moments of joy during this pregnancy as well as some of your greatest moments of grief.

Day 17

THE COURAGE TO BELIEVE
IN A MIRACLE

Is anything too hard for the Lord?
—Genesis 18:14

Perhaps nothing magnified the miracle of conception and birth more than my failed pregnancies. Through loss, I came to understand that something that had once seemed common, routine, was nothing short of extraordinary.

There are just so many intricate processes that must take place—not only to become pregnant but for a pregnancy to develop into a baby that grows and is born alive and prepared to experience life outside the womb. During pregnancy after loss, the idea that any of it—or *all* of it—might go right seemed like an extreme stretch of the imagination, one that would soon snap me back into the reality of grief. Like a rubber band that's stretched beyond its limits, my beyond-the-realm-of-possibility pregnancy just didn't seem capable of surviving the whole complicated process for long.

Today, it's hard for me to comprehend how I ever could have thought having a baby was ordinary, a given.

I was one day short of the gestational age at which Micah had been born still when an abnormality appeared during one of my routine examinations. The ultrasound showed a beating heart and a growing baby cocooned in his temporary home. Had it not been pointed out to me, the bright white spot on his abdomen wouldn't have drawn my attention at all. I was focused solely on the translucent outline of his body, head, and limbs and entranced by the rhythmic thump of his heartbeat.

"That heartbeat sounds beautiful," the technician said, before wiping the smear of gel from my belly and lending me a hand to help me transition from lying down to sitting up.

"I'll let the doctor know you're ready," she said as she opened the exam room door. "It should just be a few minutes."

I nodded, and once the door clicked shut, I traded the awkward white sheet for the comfort of the well-worn yoga pants that had unfailingly stretched right along with my belly and thighs.

Settling into the inviting cushions of the sofa that lined one wall of the room, I was half-grateful for the confirmation that my baby was alive and half-numb with uncertainty over what information the doctor would soon deliver. So often it was a combination of hopeful encouragement and dreadful concern, and I wondered what it would be this time.

Soon enough, the doctor entered the room, said hello, and briefly studied the ultrasound.

"Baby is measuring just where he should be," she said calmly. "And his heart rate is perfect."

She covered all the good news before landing on the topic of that spot on my baby's stomach.

"You've been informed about this calcium deposit, right?" she asked while pointing to the screen.

I looked at her blankly, unsure of what she was getting at. My regular doctor was out of the office, and based on the current ultrasound as well as this doctor's review of the previous two, she assumed the mysterious spot had been brought to my attention.

"No," I said, confused.

"Huh. I'm surprised it hasn't been mentioned to you, as it's been there for at least the last couple of weeks."

My eyes met hers, and like a deer in headlights, I froze in a state of bewilderment, unable to run from whatever bad news was coming at me.

"It's a calcification in the baby's stomach. It might be nothing at all, but you should know that it can sometimes be a marker for infection or chromosomal defects."

Infection remained a trigger word for me as the suspicion that one had been a contributing factor in Micah's death remained.

I didn't know what to say, which questions to ask. The doctor didn't seem terribly concerned, but the issue had been of enough importance to at least bring it to my attention.

Since I had another appointment already scheduled with my regular doctor the following week, the conversation stopped there. I was grateful for the news that my baby appeared to still be thriving, despite the variety of concerns that had been pointed out to me over the course of the past several weeks. First it was my cervix. Then sludge. Then a potential heart defect. And now calcification, with the threat of infection and genetic defects. The emergence of yet another possible complication hung in the air like spoiled fruit, and the stench of fear followed me out the door that day.

How can this end well? How is it even possible for this baby to come home? There always seems to be something considered to be abnormal. There are constant threats! How does anyone ever bring home a baby?

No longer living under the illusion that pregnancy inevitably ends well, the only thing that was clear was that it would take nothing less than a miracle to bring my baby boy home.

But day by day, that's exactly what was taking place. Every day was a series of small miracles that I hoped would end with a grand finale of me stepping out of the hospital's cool fluorescent lights and into the warm sunshine, my baby cradled in my arms and heading home with me.

Despite my doubts and the ever-present fear that gripped daily life, I clung to what I knew to be true—that nothing is too much for the God who placed a baby in my womb in the first place.

It can be hard to believe, can't it? That the baby who sleeps in your womb might one day transition to sleeping in a crib, snoring softly as you examine your miracle in vivid detail. With all you've been through—a full womb having left you empty, joy extinguished by grief—how can you be expected to believe that this time will be different? Scripture tells us that even Sarah laughed in disbelief when she overheard the news that she would give birth to a son, for she was old and had only known barrenness (Genesis 18:10–12). Yet, a year later, Isaac was born. Because God is a God of miracles. Then *and* now. The miracle you're waiting for isn't beyond his ability. After all, his very own Son was conceived in the womb of a virgin, an impossibility for anyone but an almighty God.

Like you, I know that if pregnancy after loss is anything, it's *hard*. Physically and emotionally, with the weight of it all rarely easing up. It's hard to put one foot in front of the other, believing that your pregnancy will result in a baby to nurse and soothe, one that will eventually call you Mama.

But nothing is too hard for God. Will he allow you to deliver a living child? I can't say. But he certainly *can*. The miracle of today is that there is a baby inside you. And I pray that the miracle in your womb becomes a miracle in your arms.

God, there is never a shortage of concern when it comes to my pregnancy and the future of my baby. The awareness that complications could arise at any time keeps doubt and fear at the forefront of my mind. I didn't know how common loss was until I experienced it myself. Nor did I understand the true miracle of life; how fragile it is and how intricately my body and that of my baby must work together. But now that I do, it's hard to believe that a miracle could be waiting on the other side of my pregnancy. Thank you for reminding me that you are a God of miracles. And thank you for the women who have come before me, whose bodies have birthed thriving babies when the very idea of it seemed laughable. God, I'm so grateful for the miracle of life that has taken up residence in my womb. I'm clinging to this miracle today, and even though it's hard, I'm choosing to believe that you aren't done yet. I pray that the baby in my womb will know the feeling of being cradled in my arms.

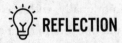 **REFLECTION**

What miracles, large or small, have you experienced during this pregnancy?

 LETTER

Tell your baby all about the miracle of his or her life up to this point in your pregnancy.

Day 18

THE COURAGE TO CREATE TANGIBLE FORMS OF HOPE

Hope deferred makes the heart sick,
but a longing fulfilled is a tree of life.
—PROVERBS 13:12

I clicked the Complete Purchase button and immediately wished I could take it back. Panic pulsed through my veins, and simply breathing took effort. I was tiptoeing toward the threshold of the third trimester, and while I'd attempted to keep my digital footsteps from leading me down the path of all things baby, the internet outmaneuvered me.

Right there on the screen flashed the most adorable set of decorative baby blocks, bearing silhouettes of woodland creatures set against the muted tones of nature. The perfect accessory for a baby boy's room.

Now I had a dilemma. I'd promised myself that I'd refrain from purchasing baby items until after my baby came home because what if he didn't? What would I do with this absolutely unnecessary set of baby blocks if I didn't actually end up with a reason to decorate a nursery? There was a chance these blocks might become objects of scorn—reminders not only of my foolishness in believing this pregnancy might work out but also of another baby who didn't survive.

But those blocks were the precise nursery accessory I didn't even know I needed. And the words *last one* and *final sale*, along with a healthy discount, stopped me in my tracks, my gaze steady as I considered how to proceed.

I can't justify spending money on something that might end up serving no purpose at all, can I?

But somehow, in that moment, the fear of missing out on this perfect set of blocks was greater than the fear of losing my baby. So I added them to my cart and quickly completed the transaction before I could change my mind.

"Congratulations on your purchase!" the screen read, failing to acknowledge that I hadn't yet accomplished the great task of birthing a living baby to whom I could give those blocks.

Immediately, my body hunched over on the stairs where I'd been sitting with my laptop. I trembled with certainty that this frivolous purchase would somehow jinx my pregnancy. The prospect of ever using what I'd just ordered seemed more like a crapshoot than cause for celebration. Soon, a package filled with building blocks of fear, hope, and skepticism would be dropped on my front porch, and tearing it open would release equal amounts of pain and possibility.

The whole thing was a distinct contrast from my very first pregnancy. The one successful pregnancy I'd had before naivete shriveled along with the fragile bodies of my next two babies. At twenty weeks pregnant with my daughter, upon finding out that she was, in fact, a girl, my husband and I had dinner out with another couple. Afterward, we separated into pairs, the women heading over to the mall to shop for baby girl clothes, leaving the men to their own devices.

Together, my friend and I selected a handful of itty-bitty frilly dresses that I couldn't wait to dress my baby girl in. They looked delicious, and holding them in my hands almost made my mouth water for the day I'd officially begin mothering her. Never did it occur to me that there was a chance she wouldn't live long enough to wear those dresses. Even though there is always a chance, I didn't really understand that then.

But I more than understood it now. A few days after my impulse purchase, the blocks arrived as expected. But the delivery made me wonder if my baby would do the same. Would he arrive as expected, or would he be lost in transit?

I tore open the package to inspect the blocks. They were even more captivating in my hands than they'd been on my screen. As I turned them between my fingers and felt the weight of them in my palms—tangible items that were specifically meant for my baby—a switch flipped in my mind, and it was as if I finally accepted that I really was pregnant.

For months, my mind had done its best to ignore what my body could not hide. Of course, I *knew* I was pregnant, but believing it and accepting it was a different story. I had remained relatively detached from the whole experience, afraid of becoming attached to a baby I wouldn't get to keep. Which is so strange because my baby had been attached to me all along.

But in that moment, those blocks somehow made my son real. I was carrying a baby. His life was being lived inside me. He really was there. And he would be born, whether alive or not. My pregnancy had been built atop the ashes of loss, and we hadn't yet escaped the danger zone, my baby and me. But those blocks? They built hope in me, despite the lingering threats.

I had purchased them with fear and trepidation vibrating in my bones, but as I clicked Add to Cart, hope surged through my heart. My fingers were performing a simple act of bravery. For just a moment, I dared to believe that there could be—and even *would be*—a place for those blocks in my life and the life of my baby.

The blocks were the first of a handful of purchases I allowed myself to make over the next few months. With each one, I prayed that my baby would one day be able to use whatever it was I was buying for him, while simultaneously wondering if I'd end up returning it.

I never could have imagined that purchasing nursery decor or onesies or a going-home-from-the-hospital outfit could be so agonizing, presenting a dilemma I hadn't previously known existed. *Should I purchase items for a baby who might not come home or pretend this baby doesn't exist by purchasing nothing?* Neither felt right. But I came to understand that each small purchase initiated a withdrawal from my bank account while making a deposit of hope in my heart.

Each purchase felt like taking a small step away from doubt and toward hopeful possibility. And scary as it was, it felt good to take those steps. No longer was I choosing to be completely ambivalent about my pregnancy. My baby was there and was coming, and while I couldn't guarantee he'd be coming home, each purchase was a choice to believe he very well could.

When you've lost a baby and become pregnant again, it never really feels like a good time to start planning for your child's future because you aren't sure there is one. But there's a whole lot in this life that we're not sure about, and I've concluded that it never hurts to dream. It never hurts to hope. It never hurts to plan for what we so desperately wish to unfold, despite having the knowledge that sometimes plans change. Sometimes it's our hopes and dreams that carry us through the hard parts of life.

So much of my pregnancy was spent preparing my heart for the worst imaginable scenario because what was the point of creating space for hope when it had no effect on the desired outcome? But even though my longing to hold another living baby had yet to be fulfilled, wasn't it enough that my longing for another pregnancy had been fulfilled? Wasn't that in itself a branch of hope—of life—that had risen up and been extended to me from the ashes of loss? There was now something where there had been nothing, and it took one small, brave step toward planning for the future of that something for me to believe that maybe, just maybe, life was waiting for me at the end of my pregnancy.

Those baby blocks were, in a way, a foundation on which my hope was built. And isn't that what faith is too? And God? Foundations on which we build our hope? We are always searching for better circumstances in this life. And while pregnancy after loss isn't exactly the way we'd hoped to experience pregnancy, isn't it enough to help us cling to God's promise of a better day? Isn't today, with your womb full, a better day than when it was so heartbreakingly empty? Hasn't faith, even the smallest amount, carried you to this point?

God has given you this child right now, and even if you can't predict what the future holds—even if you're scared and unsure and hope seems impossible to grasp—might the life that's inside you right now be enough to spur you toward embracing that elusive hope in a tangible way?

You might not be able to see your baby, but maybe his or her presence can spur you on in faith to plan, even in the smallest ways, for the future you wish your baby to have. One tiny, courageous step at a time. Then, maybe, just maybe, you'll be able to see hope and grab hold of the beauty that is even now springing up from the ashes.

God, hope is elusive right now. I see women purchasing baby clothes and scroll past images of beautiful nurseries, but it's just so hard for me to believe that there will be a place in my life for those things. I've so often brushed past hope and taken up residence in fear and anxiety because somehow that seems safer. Help me see possibility instead of pain in all things baby. I don't want to shield myself any longer from the tiny clothes and adorable decor that bring joy to other women but feel like a jinx to me. God, help me to embrace the little necessities and baby accessories. I want to see them as markers of hope, symbols of possibility. Help me to remember that while I wait for the fulfillment of the longing to hold my baby in my arms, another longing already has been fulfilled—evidenced by my growing belly and the life taking shape within me. Help me to hold fast to your promise to bring beauty from ashes.

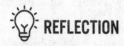 **REFLECTION**

Overall, how would you describe your feelings about tangible forms of hope, such as baby toys, clothing, and supplies? What,

if anything, keeps you from planning for your baby's arrival? If you were to take one small step toward a tangible form of hope, what would it be?

 LETTER

Tell your baby how you are planning now or how you will plan in the future for his or her arrival. What steps are you taking, even if small ones?

Day 19

FINDING PEACE IN THE FOG

The Lord himself goes before you and will be
with you; he will never leave you nor forsake you.
Do not be afraid; do not be discouraged.

—DEUTERONOMY 31:8

One morning, as I drove Annabel to school, the fog was so thick I could hardly see beyond the frame of my car. I knew where I was, but I didn't know with certainty where I was going. I couldn't even see the road—was I on it? I couldn't see vehicles, animals, or other potential obstacles, though I knew the possibility of them being near. *Should I really be doing this? Driving in this fog?*

At the same time, I also had a sense that the fog was somehow shielding us from the outside world, as if nothing could touch us. We were cocooned in the car, my daughter with her baby on her lap and me with mine in my belly. It was quiet but for the steady hum of the car's engine. Whatever distractions might have been present outside of my car were hidden by the thick wall of clouds.

In the moments before we emerged from the dense curtain of gray—before safety was fully realized—I felt a strange sense of comfort, as if what I had in that moment was enough. Me, my daughter, and my yet-to-be-born son—together. Somehow, even in the insecurity of driving in fog, I felt peace as I paid special attention to two prayers that had been answered—one in the back seat, and one in my belly.

Driving through fog is a pretty good metaphor for pregnancy after loss. We know where we are, but we can't see where we're going. We maneuver slowly through the uncertainty of pregnancy, our vision clouded, without knowing what lies ahead, beyond the haze. Even though we can't see it, we are aware of the dangers lurking all around us, and we know they could hit us head-on at any time. With all the data available about hearts that stop, genetic defects, placental abruptions, premature labor, and any other number of dangerous conditions, there is no telling if the babies we carry will come out safely on the other side.

Shortly after I dropped off Annabel at school, the fog we'd driven through cleared, revealing a baby-blue sky and sunshine so bright I wondered if its warmth could penetrate the walls of my womb.

But the fog of pregnancy after loss stuck around, always seeming to follow me.

I was still asking the same types of questions I had scratched out on paper in the church parking lot during the early weeks of my pregnancy. *Should I really be doing this? Should I really have gone this direction when it could lead to more loss? Should I really have entered this fog with no promise that I'll reach a clearing?*

Since I was already pregnant, of course I was supposed to be persisting through it. But the feeling that I wasn't really meant to be in this position in the first place lingered. I was always second-guessing my circumstances and trying to determine God's plan for my pregnancy.

Unlike the foggy quiet of the car ride that day, my mind was rarely silent. The incessant noise of worry clanged in my head like crashing cymbals in the hands of a clumsy child. I was constantly fearful of unseen dangers as I inched my way through the unknown.

I wanted the peace that came with answers, with a glimpse into the future, with a hint about what was going to happen next. But I didn't have any of those things, and I wasn't going to get them—not until my pregnancy came to an end in one way or another. But it turns out that my problem wasn't my lack of knowledge and foresight—it was that I was so focused on where I was going that I often forgot where I was.

I was pregnant, gloriously pregnant, despite the state of confusion that came with it.

If only my mind could be quieted in the fog of pregnancy just as it had been in the car on the way to school that morning. If only I could settle my anxious thoughts long enough to take inventory of what I knew to be true minute by minute. If only I could channel the peace from those moments I felt cocooned in the car, content with what I had with me even though I couldn't see what was ahead.

I didn't need all of my questions answered to accept peace, even though that's what I would have preferred. Instead of relying on certainty to surround me in a sense of calm, what I really needed was peace to shield me from the unknowns, a peace that said, *No matter what happens, you aren't driving through the fog alone.* I needed a peace anchored in the realization that what I already had was enough, even if I ended up in the ditch.

As much as we long for answers and hard facts, peace doesn't come from knowing how everything will turn out. It comes from knowing that *God* knows how everything will turn out; from knowing he is trustworthy and won't leave us alone in the fog. We might not be able to see, but he can. He knows the dangers we face, he knows where we're headed, and he's guiding us through the good and bad, even when we can't see anything.

In fact, Scripture tells us that God himself has been known to take on the form of a cloud to guide his people through perilous circumstances (Exodus 13:21). At times, the cloud itself made his presence unmistakable, his glory undeniable (Exodus 16:10). Sometimes it's when we are surrounded by our own clouds and fog that he draws closest to us, surrounding us with peace when we can't see clearly enough to navigate on our own.

We might follow behind blindly, unsure of our next steps, but through prayer, peace is not out of reach. We grab hold of it when we stop trying to figure everything out and pay attention to the prayers that have already been answered. Like the prayer about getting a positive pregnancy test. And the one about hearing your baby's heartbeat. And the one about your pregnancy surviving another day.

Friend, pregnancy after loss means we are never going to be fully confident in where pregnancy is going or what obstacles we might encounter. We can't be because we just don't know. But we do know that God goes before us and that he's weaving together each thread of our lives—even the frayed and weak ones—into a beautiful tapestry that will, in some way, be a blessing to us.

Nothing is clear in the fog, but we can find peace even there when we look down at the gift in our growing bellies and realize we aren't on this foggy road alone. We can praise God for the answered prayer of a flourishing womb and pray as we navigate the unknown, knowing that he's guiding us.

God, nothing about my pregnancy is clear. I feel like I'm inching my way through a thick fog, unable to see anything. I constantly wonder what unseen danger might threaten my baby, wishing I could see ahead to avoid whatever troubles might be near. Because I can't see what the future of my pregnancy holds, it's difficult to find peace. I want answers. I believe that if I could just get them, then I would have peace. But I also know that true peace comes only from hoping and trusting in you, from knowing you can see beyond the fog and that you're guiding me through it. Remind me that it's not certainty I need in order to find peace; it's your peace that I need to guard me from the uncertainty. God, I praise you for this baby in my womb, and I pray that you will bring us both safely through the fog.

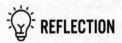 **REFLECTION**

How would you describe the fog you're navigating right now? What is it you can't see? In what ways do you need God's peace to guard your heart and your mind from the uncertainties?

 LETTER

Describe to your baby moments of comfort you've experienced, even in the unknowns of pregnancy.

Day 20

REFUGE FOR WHEN YOU ARE EXPOSED

Whoever dwells in the shelter of the Most High
will rest in the shadow of the Almighty.
I will say of the LORD, "He is my refuge and my
  fortress,
my God, in whom I trust."

—PSALM 91:1–2

Throughout my pregnancy, I secretly yearned to retreat into a state of hibernation. It wasn't realistic, I knew, but as longings often do, this one penetrated the walls of reason, planting deep roots that edged into every crevice of my body, mind, and spirit. *This would be so much easier if I could just sleep through the whole thing and wake up to a crying baby in my arms.* How wonderful it would have been to abandon the outside world and curl up in the cozy refuge of my bed and sleep for nine months straight!

I was convinced that if I could just hide from the debris of loss swirling around me—the grief, fear, skepticism, panic—everything

133

would be okay. My baby and I would both safely exit the dangerous territory of pregnancy after loss. We would escape the impending doom my restless mind was always imagining. But I never found such a hiding place. Even my doctor's office wasn't safe, though I liked to think otherwise.

"I wish I could just live here until the baby is born," I said to my doctor during an appointment. It was a thought I'd had a thousand times, and though I don't remember my exact concerns that day (because there were *always* concerns), it was all I could say to convey what I was feeling.

With its leather couches in the waiting room, essential oils dispersing pleasant aromas into the otherwise sterile air, calming background music, and, of course, ultrasound machines that so far had stifled worry, it was a place I daydreamed of calling home while pregnant. A shelter from the bitter reality of loss. I dreamed of being monitored and reassured every single day—that was the ideal. But ideal doesn't exactly exist when you're pregnant after loss. As soon as the words *pregnancy* and *loss* intermingle, *ideal* completely dissolves.

My doctor responded to my comment as if I were joking, but I meant it. I just wanted to feel safe. I wanted to hear my baby's heartbeat every second of every day, to watch him come to life on the ultrasound monitor at will—to know that he was alive!

You wouldn't think that lying on a cold exam table, body exposed and sticking to a sheet of crinkly paper, would create an atmosphere of comfort. But that table was my safe space—at least when my doctor told me what I wanted to hear.

And yet, doctor's office or not, safety was an illusion. Despite receiving mostly good news up to that point in my pregnancy, it was on similar exam tables that I had been given so much bad news. *Ectopic pregnancy. Not viable. No amniotic fluid. Termination recommended. Your baby isn't alive.* News that immediately squashed the innocent assumption that such places were safe.

Loss shifted my perspective as well as the emotions I associated with pregnancy. For many women, reaching a certain point in pregnancy—often the second trimester—is considered the point of safety. But not for the mother who has lost a pregnancy. The pure joy of pregnancy had been diluted by grief and doubt, its aftertaste bitter rather than sweet.

I was no longer a woman resting in the belief that being pregnant with a child results in parenting that child.

Sure, my health-care providers surrounded me with as many layers of protection as they could. Early appointments. Weekly cervical checks and ultrasounds. Genetic testing. Medication. Progesterone shots. In-home visits from a nurse. Collaboration between care providers. And my husband, family members, and friends offered layers of help to relieve both physical and emotional stress. They supported me by doing housework, providing meals, running errands, and providing childcare.

But while those layers of support were all good things, all useful in helping me navigate a season in which I just wanted to hide, none of them could fully protect me and my baby. Tragedy could still push its way through. An ultrasound could reveal that my baby's heart had stopped. Medication and progesterone shots were a precaution, not a guarantee. Care providers were human, not God. No matter how hard they tried or how much they wanted my pregnancy to succeed, they had limited control over the outcome. And no matter how much help I had managing my external life, there was no way of gauging its impact on the life that was growing within me.

That's the hard part, isn't it? No matter what we do or what other people do for us, we can never truly be sure that any of it will secure the results we hope for. The higher level of care, increased precautions, and extra help were good for me on so many levels, but they didn't guarantee I'd have a baby to bring home.

Friend, pregnancies that come after loss have a way of exposing us—of exposing the holes in an otherwise beautiful experience. How precious is it to carry life within our bodies? To have a womb to house our babies, becoming a vessel of life? And yet, death can still sneak in. Even our bodies are not an indestructible shelter for these cherished lives we carry.

So how do we proceed when we can't escape the knowledge that there is no truly safe place for our bodies or our babies? When we are exposed, with no shelter of absolutes or guarantees in which to rest? When this earth cannot provide the hiding place we seek?

We gather our courage to trust in God and take refuge in the shelter of his faithfulness. It's not easy. Just as pregnancy after loss takes an extraordinary amount of physical and mental energy, so does choosing to trust in God when the so-called safe zones of this world, of pregnancy, fail us.

Because what other choice is there? We know all too well the impermanence of things on this earth, the crumbling of assumptions we once perceived as certainties. We've walked in the shadow of death and destruction. But staying there will only serve to make hope disappear, tethering us to darkness and fear.

But the shadow of the Lord? That's where we find rest and peace in a layer of durable protection that this world will never provide. That's where we find refuge from the exposure of loss.

God, I often daydream about escaping my circumstances by way of a deep sleep. If I could just check out until my baby is born— until I know that he or she is going to survive the possibility of loss—my pregnancy would be so much easier. Because even when I receive assurance from doctors and help from those who love me, the shadows of loss loom, and I am reminded that nowhere is safe. God, I pray that you would give my doctors wisdom to cover me in as many layers of earthly protection as possible and that you would provide help through those who are close to me. Help me to rest in your faithfulness so that I may trust you when safe places in this world cannot be found. Help me to step out of the shadow of loss and into the shadow of the Almighty.

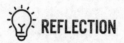

REFLECTION

What daydreams have you had about securing safety? (For example, going into hibernation or living at the doctor's office.) What thoughts or emotions come to mind when you imagine taking rest and refuge in the shadow of the Almighty instead?

LETTER

Write a letter to God in which you lay out your deepest fears and emotions regarding this season. Ask him to help you trust him and rest in his provision.

THE COURAGE TO TAKE THE PICTURE

But Mary treasured up all these things
and pondered them in her heart.

—LUKE 2:19

My experience with loss was laced with regret.

The first time it happened I had only just discovered I was pregnant, which meant I had barely begun to process the fact that I was or had been pregnant at all. But the second time? That pregnancy had continued for more than twenty weeks, and yet I had just one photo of my baby bump to show for it. I regretted that.

Prior to Micah being stillborn, intuition had put me on high alert. Early on, a hushed knowing that things were going to take a turn in the wrong direction began circulating through my body, though I couldn't pinpoint when or how it would happen. Though this feeling didn't really make sense since appointments and ultrasounds revealed nothing but a healthy baby and a normal pregnancy, I just knew something was off.

Unlike I had done in the past, I didn't make the standard second-trimester pregnancy announcement. My husband and I quietly told a few select people. Even friends I saw on a regular basis weren't informed I was pregnant until I wasn't pregnant anymore. I didn't mention it on social media or take weekly snapshots of my waistline. I took just that one snapshot, more out of obligation than celebration, and refused to treat my pregnancy as if anything were promised.

When I make it to twenty weeks, I'll make it official, public.

But one month after that photo was taken, I delivered a stillborn baby. Knowing beforehand what the fate of my baby would be, I had brought a camera, but I never took it out of my bag.

I wanted to chronicle the experience, the only time I would have with my baby in the flesh, but I was afraid to ask anyone to take pictures of labor, delivery, and the moments I spent face-to-face with Micah. I was worried about what the nurses would think. I wasn't sure what was normal or acceptable when one's baby dies. I was afraid it was too strange a request to speak aloud because isn't it morbid and perverse to photograph the makings of death?

I was grateful that the nurses took pictures of Micah with the staff camera and sent them home with me. But I have no idea where the photos were taken—somewhere in the dark recesses of the hospital morgue, I imagined. Which may not have been the case, but since it was death being photographed, I couldn't help but imagine the scene as somewhere dank and colorless.

There were no photos taken of Micah and me together. The

nurse took my baby from me and returned from an unknown place with a few glossy images.

I regret not speaking up and asking for what I so deeply wanted. For not mustering the courage to photograph those weeks in which Micah lived in my womb despite the rumblings of tragedy pulsing through me. My time with Micah was so limited, and that one baby bump photo along with the few images from the hospital just weren't enough. So much of the story was left out. I wanted an album documenting the entirety of our twenty-plus weeks together, partially to prove that my pregnancy—and Micah's life—was more than a figment of my imagination.

So, when I became pregnant again, you'd think I would have tried to avoid the inevitable regret of not taking enough pictures by taking as many pictures as possible. But no.

I underestimated how stubborn I can be. I wasn't going to slap a picture-perfect smile on my face when every single week felt like a slow, toilsome shuffle from start to finish. And it seemed inappropriate to take pregnancy pictures that highlighted the hardened facial features of a woman who was far too familiar with the grim combination of babies and death.

Just surviving from one day to the next was a true labor of love that required every bit of energy I had. I didn't have the capacity to curate inauthentic images depicting how I was supposed to be feeling. And who wants photographic evidence of being the doom-and-gloom pregnant lady?

But no one wants to live under a shroud of regret, either, which I admit is where I find myself today. Not that it's horrible or the worst thing that could happen, or that happiness hasn't found me. I just wish that when I paged through our family photo books,

I'd find happy, even if staged, memories of being pregnant with my son like I have of the pregnancy with my daughter.

The regret I so adamantly thought I would avoid still lingers as I scroll through a total of five poorly lit, grainy photos that I forced myself to take while I was pregnant after loss. It's certainly not the collection of weekly milestone photos I assumed I'd have.

What I didn't realize was just how scary it would be to allow myself to be photographed. With a lens pointed at my belly, I couldn't deny that I really was pregnant—and also really scared. It was easier to pretend there wasn't a baby growing in there than to risk the vulnerability of documenting a tiny human I could not yet see. If I fully acknowledged my baby's presence, I might become too attached. And if that happened, wouldn't that make it even harder if I lost him?

I knew I wanted photos, *really, really* wanted them. But I couldn't talk myself into contacting a local photographer when I knew it would lead to questions I didn't want to answer. *Is this your first pregnancy? How many kids do you have? Aren't you excited?* Just the thought of having to speak with a cheerful voice on the other end of the line was enough to put me off.

But God placed an opportunity in my lap when a friend told me she knew a photographer who needed a "model" to help build her maternity photo portfolio. I wasn't sure she would be satisfied with a somewhat disheveled and skeptical woman who was struggling to admit she was even pregnant. But the session was free, and all I had to do was send her an email. It was a nudge from above—something I desperately wanted but had been too scared to pursue.

I was uncomfortable the entire time. Not just because I had entered the third trimester and was quickly gaining weight but because the photo session involved more walking than I was used to as well as posing in awkward positions. I was worried I would go into labor or start bleeding or experience some other pregnancy-related mishap.

But I treasure those photos today. As hard as it was, I want to remember that I smiled, and I want my children to see that I smiled too. Even if it felt forced, my son deserved it. After loss, it truly was the most beautiful thing I could imagine, despite being perhaps the second-most taxing experience of my life.

You've probably figured out by now that I wasn't exactly a glowing example of what a pregnant woman is *supposed* to look like. But if you do anything—if you take to heart any part of this book—make it this: take the picture! Take a whole bunch of them. Pregnancy after loss can sometimes feel like trying to uncover buried treasure. You keep digging through the grief and fear in search of that glimmer of hope, that glint of life that somehow lets you know that everything will be okay. Maybe you won't find it—I pray you do—but I challenge you to keep searching and to consider that the treasure might be found in the lens of a camera.

Sometimes I think about Mary, the mother of Jesus, and how hard the circumstances surrounding her pregnancy must have been. Virgin. Unmarried. Pregnant in a society that certainly shunned such a thing, without even a decent place to birth her baby, the Savior of the world.

Yet we are told she treasured the happenings around the birth of her baby, keeping them close to her heart. Sure, this was the birth of Jesus we're talking about, but I can't help but think that this same mindset applies to our pregnancies as well. After all, Jesus was created in the womb, too, and we know a child is just as precious before birth as after.

Even during a difficult pregnancy, there is so much beauty to be appreciated. So much goodness. So much that we're going to want to remember and hang on to, even if it doesn't feel as if this is true at the time.

Maybe, like me, you're erring on the side of emotional detachment as a means of self-protection. Maybe you're scared because the grim memories aren't yet distant enough, causing you to fear that documenting your pregnancy with photos will somehow attract calamity.

But your pregnancy and your baby are worth letting down your guard.

At the risk of sounding like one of those slap-happy grandmas at the grocery store, you might not treasure the experience now (if you do, I'm truly thrilled for you), but one day I believe you will. In fact, you *might* even miss it. And I hope that, unlike me, you're without regret as you page or scroll through an album of photos to accompany the roller coaster of memories attached to your pregnancy—and your sweet baby.

God, it's no secret that I want this pregnancy to pass quickly, that I just want to fast-forward to the end, where my baby is born, so we can truly start our life together. But I also know that there is so much beauty happening in the day-to-day as I wait for my baby to be born, even though it sometimes gets lost in the stress of it all. I know I'm going to want to remember the details of this pregnancy even though I so often want to brush right past them. God, I pray for the courage to take the picture—to take lots of them—so I can remember these precious days during the very beginnings of my child's life. Help me to treasure these days instead of wishing them away.

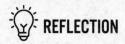

REFLECTION

What emotions are you aware of when you consider document-ing moments from your pregnancy with photos? How might taking photos benefit you now and in the future?

LETTER

Which details of your pregnancy stand out as the most memorable ones up to this point? Tell your baby about them.

Day 22

A PLACE WHERE HONESTY IS MET WITH UNDERSTANDING

But you, God, see the trouble of the afflicted;
you consider their grief and take it in hand.
—PSALM 10:14

Two days before what had been Micah's due date, I was visiting with a friend who gently broke the news that she was pregnant. I wasn't surprised, as I knew she and her husband had been trying to conceive, but the fact that she was expecting a baby when I was supposed to be welcoming mine was hard.

She was overflowing with compassion and poured so much grace over me when she said she didn't expect me to be happy for her and that it was okay if I wasn't. For that, I was grateful. I didn't feel like I deserved a pass to be upset about someone else's good news, but she gave me one anyway, and I was glad to have it.

Later that evening, Luke found me crumpled into a ball on the bathroom floor, sobbing over the unfairness of it all.

"I should be having a baby!" I wailed. "Everyone is having babies, and I'm never going to have another one!"

I cried myself to sleep that night and woke in the morning only to remember my friend's good fortune and begin another cycle of tears.

The complexity of emotions that surround pregnancy loss and life after that loss is often ignored and misunderstood. My friend and my husband were gentle with my heart, judgment-free companions who recognized deep pain and responded accordingly. But that's not always the case. People who have the ability to respond in such a way aren't always easy to find when the clouds of loss blow in and loom even after you become pregnant again.

I once had someone tell me that she was upset after her friend who'd had two miscarriages said to her, "I'm going to be so mad if you have a baby before I do." No, it's not exactly a kind statement to make, but as mothers who have lost, we can identify with how painful it is to watch other women bring babies home when our arms remain empty.

Another time, a woman confided in me that after she shared how hard it was to be pregnant after loss, someone told her to "just be grateful" she was pregnant again. *Doesn't she know that I could lose this one too?* she wondered.

In the world of loss and subsequent pregnancies, our honest feelings aren't always met with understanding, which intensifies the loneliness of these experiences.

I know that's how I felt the day after my friend delivered the news of her pregnancy. I was alone in a world that seemed hell-bent on moving forward when my life didn't seem to be moving at all.

So I did the only thing I knew to do, which was to connect in a private online group created specifically for loss moms, where I could share my honest feelings.

I don't think my husband knows what to do with me!

I feel unfit for society.

I don't think I can be a good friend, even though I want to be.

I don't want to be jealous or emotionally unstable, but I cannot stop crying.

I don't feel capable of being happy for others.

After sharing my story, I was met with a number of responses that normalized what I was feeling, at least under the circumstances.

This is something we all struggle with.

It's a normal part of the grieving process. Nothing is wrong with you.

It's okay to step back for a while if you need to.

I'd like to say that typing out my feelings changed how I felt, that my emotions evolved into something a little more socially acceptable after I became pregnant again, but I'd be lying. Because the experiences of pregnancy loss and pregnancy after loss are so intricately tied together that many of the same emotions are going to be wrapped around both.

Online support groups—ones that safeguarded the secrets of loss moms—were a safe haven for my troubled thoughts and complicated emotions. Especially during my subsequent pregnancy, when I felt the unspoken pressure to "just be grateful." When I didn't fit the image of the blissfully pregnant woman. When I couldn't live up to the expectations of what pregnancy is supposed to look like. When I could hardly even admit I was pregnant.

There, the things that others seemed incapable of comprehending were accepted, understood. The words that brought the greatest comfort—*me too*—had never been in greater supply. No one expected me to clean up my emotions or to soak them up with a platitude, gratitude, or positive attitude just because I was pregnant again.

After my first loss, I had felt misunderstood in my grief among the non-grieving, and those feelings compounded times ten when I was pregnant after loss. It was such a relief to have a safe place among other women who understood. Within a community of loss moms, we could all discuss how we felt with people who didn't glibly promise that our babies would be okay or treat our pregnancies as if they hadn't arisen out of the worst circumstances.

We heard the heartbeat today. I'm grateful but still an anxious mess. I think I have food poisoning. The worry never ends.

Made it to twenty-four weeks. Still extremely anxious but grateful to have made it this far.

I'm being induced in three weeks, and the last several days I've had an absolute feeling of dread.

It sounds silly, but I'm worried my baby is moving too much.

There continues to be a part of me that feels my baby is safer on the outside than on the inside, even though I'm only thirty-three weeks.

It was a community of true solidarity. A place where we lamented with one another but also celebrated. Because when a fellow loss mom shares her success story and photos of her baby born after loss, alive and well, it's like receiving a pure dose of hope. Real hope instead of the false hope that so easily rolls off the tongues of those who haven't lost a baby.

As much as we want to be understood, people are sometimes going to fail us. In a perfect world, our concerns and feelings regarding our subsequent pregnancies would be met only with understanding and compassion. But if this were a perfect world, we wouldn't be pregnant after loss. We'd simply be pregnant. Gleefully, obliviously pregnant.

If you don't necessarily feel supported in the way you need to be—if your honesty is mistaken for ingratitude—it's okay to seek solace in places where the phrase *me too* is more common than platitudes such as "everything will work out." It's okay to find a safe place where your honesty is met with help and hope instead of responses that hurt, even if unintentionally. It's okay to surround yourself with those who get it.

Maybe that safe place is an online group filled with other women who can relate to what you are experiencing. It might be a local grief-support group that meets face-to-face. Or maybe it's a mental health professional who specializes in grief, pregnancy loss, and pregnancy after loss—you can ask your health-care provider for recommendations and a referral.

Whatever form the support takes, we weren't meant to endure this season alone. We need those who have been there to help us, to lift us up with their shared experiences, to help us feel seen and understood. We need empathy and a safe place to lament.

> Two are better than one,
>> because they have a good return for their labor:
> If either of them falls down,
>> one can help the other up. (Ecclesiastes 4:9–10)

There might be times when you feel judged or misunderstood when bravely admitting how you're *really* doing. When that happens, remember that our sovereign God isn't judging you for your grief and trepidation. He understands that you'll be impacted by the brokenness of this world and of your life. He understands how much it weighs on you, and he doesn't ask you to gloss over it like people sometimes do. He understands the affliction that arises from loss. He understands that pregnancy after loss is unspeakably hard and acknowledges that it was never supposed to be this way.

> Then you will call on me and come and pray to me, and I will listen to you. (Jeremiah 29:12)

When you feel alone, cry out to him. Describe your fear. Ask for relief. Beg him to let you keep this baby. He sees all of you and is listening with an open heart and pure intentions that only a perfect God can have.

While my husband, my friend, and those women in my online support groups held so much of my grief, God was no doubt holding my hurt and heartache in full. Where people lacked capacity to see and support me, God surely did not. And I believe with all my heart that he is doing the same for you.

> *God, it really bothers me when people brush aside my hurt and mistake my honesty for ingratitude. You know I am grateful for this baby I'm carrying, but you also know this pregnancy is complicated. Thank you for allowing me to lament. I trust that you are not judging me for grieving and groaning. Please guide me toward a safe community in which I can be honest about the hardships surrounding my pregnancy. I crave empathy and solidarity with others who can fully understand me. When people say the wrong thing, help me to respond in grace and turn to you for comfort, realizing humans aren't perfect and hurtful words are often unintentional. It's hard to explain that this pregnancy is both an affliction and a blessing, but I know you understand.*

I cry out to you with my fears. I ask that you provide relief. And again, I'm begging you to let me bring this baby home.

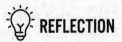 REFLECTION

How do you tend to respond when people say things about your loss and subsequent pregnancy that hurt, even if unintentionally? In what ways, if any, do you wish you could respond differently?

 LETTER

Write a letter to the people who don't understand. What honest—if not always easy to admit—feelings around being pregnant after loss would you share to help them understand?

Day 23

THE COURAGE TO SHAMELESSLY DEPEND ON GOD

Is anyone among you in trouble? Let them pray.

—JAMES 5:13

I dropped Annabel off at preschool and returned home to rest on the couch until it was time to pick her up. With my hand resting on my belly, I prayed the same prayer I'd prayed no less than a thousand times.

God, please let him kick. Please, God. Let. Him. Kick. Please.

And then that sweet baby boy kicked with a vigor that was hard to imagine coming from a tiny being who couldn't have weighed more than a pound or two.

I counted kicks and punches and tumbles while continuing to pray. *Thank you, God. Thank you. Thankyouthankyouthankyou.* Tears of relief welled in the corners of my eyes—not with enough force to make their way down my cheeks, but with enough weight to remind me that my ability to feel pure joy was still in there, still able to rise from the depths of a tumultuous pregnancy.

In that moment, joy was buoyed by the unmistakable evidence of life within, floating comfortably on the surface of my pregnancy where the presence of my baby could, in that moment, be confirmed.

When I retrieved my little girl from the school playground later that morning, I avoided eye contact with the other moms lest they perceive an inadvertent glance as permission to make conversation about my pregnancy. Despite my answered prayer a short time earlier, I couldn't be certain that it would be answered again. I couldn't even be certain that it meant my baby was still alive by the time I stepped foot on that playground. And without that certainty, I had no interest in discussing pregnancy as it's so often talked about in circles of women—with confidence of what is to come and with the presumption that pregnancy ends with innocent life rather than heart-stopping death. Whatever confidence I might once have had was six feet under with the baby I'd buried. And just like that baby, my innocence no longer existed.

I felt like such a pitiful creature. Unfit for society. In need of constant reassurance. Incapable of talking about pregnancy. Unable to cope through use of deep breathing and optimistic mantras. I wanted so desperately to "look on the bright side," but my pregnancy had so much darkness surrounding it that whatever bright side there was at any given moment still appeared rather dim.

People saw a pregnant woman and assumed the best. But they couldn't see the constant tug-of-war between the flicker of hope and the flames of devastation. I remained somewhere in the middle of that tug-of-war, never sure which direction I was going to be pulled in.

I spent my days lifting up a continuous cycle of distressed prayers to God, feeling completely inadequate in knowing that, try as I might, there really wasn't much more I could do.

I have to think that all moms pray over their unborn babies. I know I did during my first pregnancy. I prayed for a healthy baby. I prayed she would be well taken care of even though I had no idea what I was doing. I prayed she would know what a good mom was and that somehow, in all my inadequacy, I would be one to her. I prayed God would take care of her while she was inside me, still out of reach. But at that time, my prayers weren't of the on-my-knees-begging type. They were more of the fall-asleep-halfway-through type because of course a mother prays for her child.

But after a certain point in pregnancy, what was there to pray for? Back then, I didn't believe something could go wrong. Not after that first twelve or thirteen weeks. I don't even think I considered it. Because back then, I believed that control was something I could, to some extent, grab hold of. All I had to do was eat the right foods, stay out of hot tubs, and transfer litter box duty to my husband. And of course, visit my OB every now and then.

But when you do all the right things and still lose your baby, you realize how little control you actually have. When I became pregnant after losing Micah, I again did all the right things but knew that nothing I did or didn't do could guarantee the result I hoped for. Really, I couldn't depend on much of anything. Not my body. Not my good decisions. Not modern medicine. Not a book that promised to let me in on the secrets of what to expect when I was expecting.

Sure, I made decisions based on the best interests of my unborn baby, but even then, what else could I actually rely on other than

God? I didn't know what his answers to my prayers would be, but in a season of unknowing, the only thing I knew for sure was that he was really all I had.

I quickly learned that no mom prays over her unborn baby more than a mom who is pregnant after loss. This time, my prayers weren't out of obligation but desperation. I made no assumptions. I was fully aware of the possibility that even the most ideal circumstances surrounding my pregnancy might not be enough. Not only did I understand my pregnancy *could* end at any time, I believed there was a good chance it *would*.

The only thing I could control was my response to my obvious lack of control, which was often to simply be still and pray. So I prayed like my baby's life depended on it. I prayed every second of every day. Really, I did. Even when I was speaking to another human being, my brain was still churning out prayer, a silent, ongoing conversation between me and God.

Let him be okay. Please, God. Let him move. Thank you for this baby. Keep him alive until my next appointment, God. Please. Don't let there be any blood. Let me keep this one. I love him, God. Don't make me say goodbye to another one. Should I call the doctor, God? Is something wrong, or am I just paranoid? Thank you for letting me be his mom. Protect this child. Protect my heart. Carry me through this pregnancy. I can't do it without you, God. I need you. Thank you. Help.

On and on it went.

It was interesting how my prayers evolved between my first pregnancy and what would turn out to be my final one. No longer did I feel the need to pray for wisdom on how to mother the child I was carrying—that would come later, if and when it was needed. By that time, I felt confident I would be a good mom, or at least an adequate one. It's just that I didn't know if this baby would live.

That was the first order of business, which became the focus of my prayer life—that my baby boy would simply live. That I'd be given the wisdom to recognize signs of trouble. That we would know each other. That we'd both feel the comfort of my arms wrapped around him. The rest—those other prayers—I'd save them for later.

To be honest, I sometimes felt shame for my shortcomings. I saw how other pregnant women carried themselves—confident, glowing, cheerful—and felt that I was failing to live up to those traits. I wasn't strong enough, happy enough, optimistic enough, excited enough, hopeful enough. I simply wasn't enough.

But the truth is, no pregnant woman is, whether she's undeniably optimistic or trudging through pregnancy with ankles cuffed by chains of pessimism. It simply took being crushed by the devastation of loss for me to realize that.

There was no shame in stepping back, choosing stillness, and relying heavily on prayer—and on God. Nor was there shame in resting and choosing to keep to myself more than I otherwise might have. Like any woman who has experienced loss, I was still feeling my way through the aftermath. Troubled by what was behind me and by what might lie ahead.

Which is exactly when God wants us to pray. When we are in trouble—when the experience of loss both lingers and looms—this is the time to set down the weight of expectations and fold our hands in prayer. The time to rely on the power of God is precisely when we know so intimately how little power we have—regardless of what other people think.

I don't know for sure, friend, but I wonder if you're feeling even the slightest bit of shame over your weakness during this pregnancy. Over not handling the difficulty of it as well as you hoped or meeting the expectations that others have set for you. I imagine that you are raising up anguished pleas to the God of the universe, begging him for help, pleading for him to let your baby live outside your womb. Maybe you wish you felt stronger or were carrying on with life as a pregnant woman who has not experienced loss. Or maybe you're doing everything you can to control the outcome of your pregnancy but have yet to be satisfied.

It's okay to set it all aside and depend solely on God. That's what he invites us to do when trouble coils itself around us. The voice of our culture shouts "independence" and "positivity" when we're searching for hope amid the fire. But God simply invites us to pray.

He doesn't ask us to perform under the facade of being *fine*. He doesn't tell us to pretend we've got it all under control. He doesn't demand that we put on a mask of confidence, beaming from ear to ear. He tells us that we're going to struggle. He fully acknowledges that this life is trouble. And he tells us we can come to him at any time when we're in the midst of it.

God knows that pregnancy after loss is more of a trek through the wilderness than a walk in the park. And he knows that we desperately need him. Which is why he extends to us an open invitation to pray. He wants to hear from us at all times!

Pray continually. (1 Thessalonians 5:17)

He knows we can't depend on anything else in this world, so he invites us to depend on him. We know he hears us. We know he cares. We know he doesn't expect this process to be pretty or easy for us. And we know that there is no shame in depending on the God who formed the life within us.

God, sometimes I feel so pitiful, so weak during a time when I think I should be strong. Sometimes I feel ashamed by my lack of confidence and the fact that I'm not like so many of the pregnant women I'm surrounded by. I want to be able to control my situation, my pregnancy. But I can't. Help me to remember that you understand the troublesome situation I'm in and that there is no shame in depending on you. After all, there is nothing else I can depend on! Even so, I sometimes feel embarrassed by the amount of begging and pleading I do. Thank you for reminding me that you want me to pray and that there is no reason to be embarrassed by my neediness. Thank you that I don't have to perform or pretend with you. As I always do, I pray that you would sustain this sweet life within me. Thank you for letting me be this baby's mother. And thank you for always hearing my prayers.

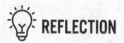

REFLECTION

In what ways are you carrying shame about your neediness or any other aspect of your pregnancy? What, if anything, keeps you from turning to God in prayer?

LETTER

Write down your prayers and your pleas for your pregnancy and your baby in a letter to God. Allow yourself to be raw as you speak to him. He is listening.

Day 24

UPROOTING THE SEEDS OF GUILT

Therefore, there is now no condemnation
for those in Christ Jesus.

—ROMANS 8:1 CSB

"Congratulations," a fellow churchgoer whispered as I approached the building's exit one Sunday morning. It was somewhere around the midpoint of my pregnancy, and while I'd attempted to disguise the extra weight I was carrying with billowy tops and bulky jackets, the charade was up. The only person I was fooling was myself. I was pregnant and well past the point of being able to cover it up.

"I thought I'd done a better job of hiding it," I whispered back, my eyes revealing a combination of surprise and unease.

"Oh, I've known for a long time," she said with a giggle. "I'm so happy for you!"

Though I couldn't match her enthusiasm, I thanked her and hurried to the car before anyone else had a chance to strike up a conversation about the pregnancy I thought I was doing such a good job of hiding.

And do you know how I felt as I drew the seat belt across my baby belly? Guilty.

Guilty for not wanting to talk about it. Guilty for not being as excited as the woman who'd congratulated me. Guilty for even trying to hide the existence of my baby in the first place. And these are just a few examples of the many ways guilt was scattered across my pregnancy like dandelion seeds in the wind.

I felt guilty for not being the shining example of a joyful pregnant woman that I thought I should be, especially since I knew how fortunate I was to actually be pregnant and to at least have the chance to have another baby. In all honesty, I felt guilty just for being pregnant because I knew there were so many women who wanted to be in my position but weren't. And then there was the guilt for focusing more on the baby I was carrying than the ones I had lost, as if putting so much energy into the baby who still had a chance at life outside my womb somehow betrayed the memory of the babies who didn't.

I felt guilty that I wasn't walking through my fourth pregnancy in the same lighthearted anticipation I'd had during my first. I hadn't even kept track of which type of fruit my baby's size resembled from week to week.

But it didn't stop there. Those seeds of guilt were scattered over other aspects of life too.

I wasn't the mom I imagined I'd be, though it was also true that I was in a season of life I hadn't imagined I'd be in. Intense grief and a complicated pregnancy hadn't been part of my plan, but those things became my reality and affected the way I parented my daughter. Sometimes I was so overcome with grief or panic that Annabel spent much of the day watching TV, getting little quality interaction from me. Other times, I said no to playdates or other kid-friendly activities because I didn't have the emotional bandwidth or physical stamina to participate. And still other times I relied on babysitters or friends and family to care for my daughter when, as her mother, I thought I should be able to do it all myself.

I felt guilty because I perceived that I was responsible for wrongdoing, that I wasn't living up to the standards of how a pregnant woman was supposed to be conducting herself. *I should be doing this. I should be feeling that. But I'm not.* The constant barrage of shoulds and my failure to follow through on them made me feel as if I were doing something wrong, as if God were pointing his finger at me in condemnation for all my shortcomings, which in turn sowed those seeds of guilt.

But the truth is, it was not God but Satan who was condemning me, causing the guilt to take root. Because the shoulds didn't take into account that this wasn't a normal pregnancy. These weren't normal circumstances. There's nothing normal about babies dying, and there's nothing normal about life after loss.

Simply put, I wasn't the same woman I'd been before loss.

I was different. Along with the new normal that we often talk about after losing a baby, there was a new normal regarding pregnancy itself, which included emotions that didn't exist before loss, as well as physical limitations. This was not wrongdoing; it was simply my reality.

I think we've been conditioned to believe that we are always supposed to be happy; that we are never supposed to struggle (or at least never admit it) or ask for help. In a do-it-yourself culture that celebrates success and promotes pleasure, it's easy to forget that hardship, tears, and grief are very normal parts of life that often require assistance from others. Life on earth includes seasons of sadness as well as joy. We experience laughter and crying, sometimes in the same breath. And our capabilities often depend on our circumstances—sometimes we knock it out of the park and sometimes we sit on the bench.

For much of my pregnancy, I assumed the latter position. Benched. I participated in life from the sidelines. I was still healing, fragile, and unable to play the game of life as actively as I once had.

And that was okay.

Because slowing down and taking care of my body was necessary for the well-being of my baby and myself too. I was tending to two vulnerable lives, and it wasn't wrong to give the needs of my unborn baby extra attention. I was juggling grief, a difficult pregnancy, and motherhood all at once, and I needed help. It surely wasn't wrong to ask for some. I was grieving two losses and carrying the possibility of a third. Certainly, lament was an acceptable response. My fourth pregnancy was not the same as my first—it came packaged with a dark history. So why did I think it *should* be the same?

Friend, false guilt can come at us from every angle during pregnancy after loss. Nothing is off-limits. Your seeds of guilt might look different from mine, but the source is the same. Satan. He loves to use shoulds to root us deep in guilt, to shame us, to point out how we're not living up to the cultural standards that have been set forth for us.

But we don't have to live up to those standards, nor do we have to live in shame. We don't have to pretend that emotional pain doesn't exist or that pregnancy after loss is easy. We don't have to feel pressured to do it all ourselves or to navigate this season perfectly. God knows we are in the trenches. He knows the depth of our grief. And when we're under attack, the only thing we really *should* do is look to him and his Word. We can uproot guilt by meditating on the truth that in him there is no condemnation, especially when we're harboring false guilt.

We don't have to let Satan's false accusations bury us. God knows our hurt, and we are allowed to feel it. He also knows our heart, which can easily fall prey to Satan's schemes—like the one in which he twists gratitude for conceiving another baby after loss into guilt, as if our pregnancy somehow exists at the expense of someone else's (reminder: it doesn't). The good news is that God is greater than all of this—our hurt, our hearts, and especially Satan.

> If our hearts condemn us, we know that God is greater than our hearts, and he knows everything. (1 John 3:20)

And with that, we are free from the guilt of the shoulds and the guilt of imperfection (perfection doesn't even exist in our human state). Free from the expectations of how we're supposed to feel or deal with the various obstacles that pregnancy after loss entails.

God, this pregnancy is not how I imagined pregnancy would be—at least before I knew what it was like to lose one. There are so many things I think I should be doing and feeling, like being more excited, planning for my baby's future, expecting the best outcome, and taking care of my other responsibilities on my own. I carry so much guilt for not walking through this season the way I think I should. Sometimes I feel guilty just for being pregnant, even though I know this child is a gift from you. I admit that I often sin, God, and for that I confess. But when I succumb to false guilt and the devil's schemes—specifically surrounding loss and pregnancy after loss—please remind me that you are greater. Help me to allow your truth to uproot the seeds of guilt and release me from the shoulds that seem to plague me.

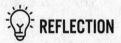

REFLECTION

What seeds of guilt have been scattered over your pregnancy? For each one, consider what it might mean that God knows everything and is greater than your heart. What, specifically, does God understand about your circumstances, about your heart?

LETTER

Counter false guilt with gratitude by telling your baby all the things for which you are thankful regarding this pregnancy.

Day 25

THE COURAGE TO CELEBRATE
EACH MILESTONE

For the Spirit God gave us does not make us timid,
but gives us power, love and self-discipline.
—2 TIMOTHY 1:7

I thought you'd feel more confident, more comfortable by now," my perinatologist said, surprised by my sullenness even after a favorable ultrasound had breathed hope into me. I'd heard the swift pumping of my baby's heart and even witnessed what looked like a *hello* wave with his tiny hand. There wasn't one bit of troubling news. And still, my expression remained grim.

She considered the appointment a milestone, as I was nearly thirty weeks into my pregnancy without major incident, and she felt comfortable releasing me from her care. Things were progressing normally, and from a medical standpoint, this doctor whom I'd seen almost weekly couldn't come up with a good reason to continue our appointments. I, on the other hand, had numerous reasons for wanting to continue under her care—the biggest being the comfort of weekly ultrasounds. But she assured me that everything was as it should be and released me into the sole care of my midwife. Yes, there had been a number of vague and undetermined concerns throughout my pregnancy, but none of them had developed into anything more. Not yet, anyway.

And that was the barrier between me and those feelings of comfort and confidence that my doctor had expected. The *not yet*. It's what had been holding me back from celebrating much of anything.

I was pregnant, but there wasn't a baby. *Not yet*. I *was* going to have a baby, but I didn't know my baby's fate upon his arrival into the world. *Not yet*. I was carrying life, but it hadn't been delivered. *Not yet*.

For months I wondered if there would be anything to celebrate. My pregnancy was a work in progress, and why would I celebrate when I wasn't yet holding the finished product?

Don't get me wrong. Throughout each and every day, I thanked God for my baby and for the gift of pregnancy. Each morning when I woke up without noticing signs of distress, I thanked him. Each time I went to the bathroom and didn't discover blood, I thanked him. With each nudge from the inside of my womb, I thanked him. But I wanted proof that my baby would survive my body, and I didn't have it. *Not yet*.

My arms could only rest on my belly, not yet able to show off a cherub for the world to see. And with over ten weeks to go, my body had not yet put the finishing touches on the form being created within it. To put it simply, this baby wasn't finalized. My pregnancy wasn't done. The comfort, confidence, and celebration would come upon completion.

I had my sights set completely on the end result, practically holding my breath while waiting to wrap my arms around my baby instead of my belly. But what if I never got to do that? Wouldn't my heart have been better served by choosing to focus on the *right now* instead of the *not yet*? Because the truth was that there were plenty of *right now* moments that had come and gone without notice. Small milestones stacked one atop another to construct what I hoped would become the ultimate milestone—the birth of a living, breathing baby who'd eventually call me Mama.

So while I was not yet gazing at my child face-to-face, while I could not yet declare victory over the battle of pregnancy after loss, while I did not yet have the proof that this pregnancy would end differently than my previous two, I *did* still have my baby. And based on previous experience, it was no small feat to be able to say that when my previous two pregnancies had never even reached the third trimester.

My baby was still a work in progress, but he was there, inside my womb. And while my eyes had been laser focused on the ultimate milestone—my son's *hopefully* normal and healthy birth—there were so many other milestones I'd let slip by without proper recognition.

For months, I told myself, *I'll celebrate when* _____. *When I make it to eighteen weeks and my water hasn't broken like it did with Micah. When I make it to twenty weeks and there are no signs of premature labor. When I reach twenty-four weeks and my pregnancy is officially considered viable. When I enter the third trimester.* But I never really did. Because each time I reached one of those milestones, my feet stayed planted in the *not yet*, and the point at which I'd allow myself to celebrate got pushed a little further out.

By this time in my pregnancy, I'd seen the beauty of a positive pregnancy test (or five). I'd landed with medical providers who collaborated, were compassionate, whom I trusted, and who did what they could to ease my distress. I'd learned sooner than I knew possible that I was growing a little boy. I'd heard his heartbeat on multiple occasions. I'd seen the growing parts of his body almost weekly. Thanks to three-dimensional ultrasound images, I'd observed his features in great detail, enough to notice his resemblance to his big sister. I'd felt his kicks. He'd survived the vulnerability of the first trimester, increased levels of cortisol due to my heightened anxiety and a number of pregnancy scares. He'd made it past viability and had entered the third trimester. He was real and he was still there.

Each one was a milestone worth recognizing precisely because each was a normal part of pregnancy that, by itself, wasn't out of the ordinary. After you've experienced the abnormal—when your womb has been a graveyard—the ordinary parts of pregnancy become extraordinary. When you're pregnant after loss, normal is a milestone worthy of celebration.

And when I really think about it, isn't every day of pregnancy after loss a milestone?

Each day of growth, change, progress toward the completion of the finished product—this is not something to brush aside in anticipation of something greater. The everyday work of pregnancy after loss is vital to completion of the project. It's difficult and draining. It includes sweat and tears, a sore body and aching heart, and an obscene amount of emotional labor. But surviving from one day to the next, waking each morning to a kicking baby, even though the worry over the life inside you threatens to suck the life out of you? This is an incredible achievement!

With progress as slow as it is, it's easy to wonder if it even matters. If the everyday moments—the small things leading up to the big reveal—even matter.

Rest assured, *they do*.

Brick by brick, day after day, the everyday moments are critical to the construction of a growing tower of milestones—of progress—that you hope and pray will be completed with the one moment you've been waiting for. The safe arrival of your baby.

Friend, I know it's hard to be enthusiastic about much of anything when you're standing in the *not yet*. How can you when you know the big moment you're waiting for might not come? When you aren't sure if your pregnancy will end with life or death?

I understand.

It takes courage to allow yourself to celebrate the *right now*—whether that's a positive pregnancy test, a weekly milestone, a kick, the powerful sound of a little heartbeat, the release to a lower level of care because pregnancy is going well, or the simple yet complicated fact that your baby is still here in a pregnancy that's progressing. Because you know it doesn't guarantee a favorable outcome. But allowing yourself to observe and honor these moments while your baby is still under construction creates space to breathe, hope, and praise God for what you do know rather than focusing solely on what you don't.

Even when you are scared, your faith gives you the power to set aside timidity, to celebrate in some small way the milestones of *right now*, even when your heart is steeped in resistance. It allows you to display the deep love for your baby through action, even if that action is small or unrecognizable to others.

I can do all this through him who gives me strength.
(Philippians 4:13)

Keep a running list of triumphs, whether big or small. Honor the progress you and your baby have made together by purchasing a meaningful gift for yourself or for your baby. Make a halfway-to-your-due-date cake and indulge in as much of it as you want. Include your husband and/or living children in the excitement of this baby's movement within you, and celebrate the evidence of this little life together. Text a friend with updates and progress and give her the opportunity to celebrate for you when you're weary. And I'll say it again: take as many photos of milestone moments (whether big or small) as your heart will allow—I promise you can't have too many.

And even in the *not yet*, free your heart to praise God for the milestones of *right now*. Without them, you wouldn't be here, in this place, with your precious baby.

God, thank you for this child I'm carrying. It might not be obvious to others, but I hope you know how grateful I truly am. My heart overflows with love for this baby, and yet I also feel heavy and burdened. It's difficult to feel joy or celebrate my pregnancy when I'm still standing in the "not yet." When I'm not sure if my baby's birth will bring life or death. I keep thinking that I'll allow myself to celebrate when I know for sure how my pregnancy will turn out. But there have been so many milestones—moments I've prayed to experience—that have come and gone without joy and celebration. God, thank you for these moments. The positive pregnancy test, the sound of a heartbeat, the weeks that have progressed into months, and more. Help me to savor these milestones by recognizing how precious they are. God, I pray for the courage to walk toward the arrival of my baby with faith, hope, and love in action.

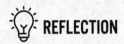 **REFLECTION**

*What moments or milestones have you experienced as you move toward the birth of your baby? List as many as you can think of. Which did you celebrate and which did you overlook? How might you celebrate the **right now**?*

 LETTER

Share with your baby the milestones that you've already accomplished and the ones you hope to experience together in the days ahead.

Day 26

CASTING OUT BITTERNESS WHEN CASUAL COMMENTS HURT

*Get rid of all bitterness, rage and anger, brawling
and slander, along with every form of malice. Be
kind and compassionate to one another, forgiving
each other, just as in Christ God forgave you.*

—Ephesians 4:31–32

I hadn't noticed it before, but being pregnant while still grieving the loss of the baby from my previous pregnancy made me
acutely aware of the casual manner in which people sometimes
speak of pregnancy. Not only was it often discussed in absolute
terms (pregnancy = baby), but it was talked about nonchalantly,
as if there were nothing more to be concerned with than minor
inconveniences.

Magazine covers and online pregnancy forums were littered
with disparaging comments and a general tone of disgust about
weight gain and postpartum bodies. Newly pregnant women

expressed disappointment in the widely accepted recommendations to refrain from drinking alcohol and eating certain foods. Ads for fitness programs made promises to help me *get my body back* after pregnancy because, apparently, the postpartum body was something to be loathed. Memes about pregnant women having to sacrifice wine or caffeine blasted my social media feed. Commercials assured me that the right cream would remove the unsightly stretch marks left behind from growing a human inside my body. Even at prenatal appointments, I occasionally saw women wearing T-shirts that proclaimed how much they missed wine or sushi.

To me, it all fell under the umbrella of complaining about things that didn't much matter. Such inconveniences and bodily changes were the last thing on my mind.

Unlike my first pregnancy, I cared nothing about how much weight I gained during pregnancy or how much of it might stick around after. I would gladly have welcomed stretch marks to consume my entire body if it meant I could also welcome a baby into this world. I wish I could say that the only things I missed were wine and sushi, but I was craving so much more.

I wanted the babies I'd lost. I wanted a normal pregnancy, unmarred by grief. I wanted to have missed the memo that sometimes babies die. I wanted my only concern to be how I'd make it through the day without a relaxing glass of wine. I wanted to be able to laugh at the blithe jokes made about pregnancy, but I no longer found there to be anything funny or casual about it.

While other pregnant women seemed willing to give anything to satisfy their taste buds with forbidden food and drink, I was willing to sacrifice everything to satisfy my aching arms with a wide-eyed baby. And I wasn't complaining about it.

On one particular Sunday, while waiting for the church service to begin, a man in the row ahead of us turned around to make small talk with Luke and me.

"Are you over it yet?" he asked. Before I had a chance to answer, he eagerly informed me that his wife had just given birth to their fourth child, but she was "over the whole pregnancy thing" by the time she was pregnant with their second. He spoke of pregnancy as if it were a drag. While I certainly wasn't enjoying every moment of mine, his words caused the seeds of resentment in my heart to bloom into full-blown bitterness.

I might have forced myself to congratulate him on the most recent addition to his family if I'd thought I could do it without bursting into tears. But tears were already threatening to spill from the corners of my eyes, so instead I pressed my lips together, forced a rigid smile, and willed myself to contain the droplets of anger and sorrow that were trying to force their way out of me.

The service started and ended with his comments that morning because even though worship began and the pastor took the stage to preach, I was not there. I sat through the service but didn't hear a word that was sung or spoken after that initial interaction. I was tossed into panic mode, unable to move for fear I would collapse if I tried, waiting for the blessing that signified the service's end so I could escape. I hated the fact that this man's wife had the privilege of casually complaining about her pregnancies. And I hated that I'd had to hear about it.

As I sat there wondering how I was going to get through the next hour, the pregnant women and babies who were present seemed to be closing in on me. I felt smothered by the awareness that they belonged and I somehow didn't. I despised being the only pregnant woman in that room without a smile and a glow.

That man's words and the presence of the smiling pregnant women hurt me and only amplified the feeling that I didn't quite fit in. My pregnancy was difficult and uncomfortable, far from the pleasurable feelings with which I'd once associated it.

Yes, I was over the fear, the anxiety, the endless tears. I was over the fact that time was moving more slowly than it ever had before. I was over coming into contact with cheery pregnant women I felt so far removed from.

But I wasn't over "it." I wasn't over being pregnant with a baby I'd prayed for with the force of a Category 5 hurricane. I felt fortunate to be noticeably pregnant because it meant that for all that had gone wrong in the past, something was going right now. It was beyond difficult, but I'd suffer endlessly to ensure my baby would have the best possible chance at life on this earth. If that meant forging ahead in discomfort and setting aside things I wanted or enjoyed, I would.

I'm willing to bet you've been the recipient of your unfair share of hurtful, inconsiderate, and misguided comments regarding pregnancy, though they were likely spoken with good intentions.

Well-meaning people see life protruding from your abdomen but not the loss that came before. Your growing bump can't convey that it is the result of a void you wish you didn't have to live with. You appear to be an average pregnant woman because no one who is pregnant after loss wears a T-shirt that says "I miss my baby who died" or "I miss being blissfully unaware that I might not get to keep this one."

And because of that, people can be reckless with their words, often because they simply don't know better. There aren't magazines in the checkout line intended for brokenhearted and scared pregnant women who are actually drawing much-needed hope from the layers of extra weight they're carrying and the stretch marks carved into their skin. Because the aftermath of loss is an invisible ailment for the woman who becomes pregnant again, society fails to recognize that many pregnancies exist beneath a veil of grief; that the potential for consequences is greater than changes in appearance or temporary inconveniences.

All of this can easily cause bitterness to rise up within us.

We want our minds to be at ease. We want to be able to travel lightly through pregnancy, but instead we're weighed down by the heaviness of heartache and crippling doubt.

Feel your feelings, friend. Acknowledge your hurt and hardship. Cry out to God at the unfairness of it all. But do not let bitterness plague your heart or your pregnancy. You have enough legitimate problems on which to expend your limited energy.

We may not always be met with grace and our pregnancy may not always be approached in the delicate manner it deserves. But we are called to give grace to others—even when they fail us—just as it's been given to us. We are called to forgive just as we've been forgiven, even when others don't know they've acted in such a way that requires forgiveness.

I don't know how to make any of this less messy, but I do know that people are going to fail us. They are going to say things that cause tears to fall and fists to clench. They aren't going to recognize the invisible pain that is an inescapable part of pregnancy after loss. But bitterness in response to these things is not going to serve us well. It will only distance us further from hope.

Praise be to the God and Father of our Lord Jesus Christ,
the Father of compassion and the God of all comfort.
(2 Corinthians 1:3)

Words hurt. But where people lack compassion, God does not. Where people fail, God does not. Where people turn a blind eye to your struggle, God does not. You can trust him to hold space for you and the inevitable mess of emotions.

It's never easy to free your heart of bitterness, but something that has helped me is remembering that loss and pregnancy after loss are experiences that can't truly be understood unless one has experienced them personally. I know that *I* haven't always been attuned to the complex nature of loss and life after loss because I didn't know better. I can even recall callous comments I've made without realizing it to those who had experienced loss and to pregnant women because I lacked understanding at the time.

Yet, despite my callousness, I received grace. And because of that, I can pass on grace to the next person who doesn't understand the pain their words have caused.

God, I've been hurt by the careless words and messages swirling around me. During a time when I need compassion and understanding, so often I haven't received it. I feel insulted when pregnancy is talked about as if it's a joke. When I'm the recipient of insensitive comments, the seeds of bitterness begin to sprout and take root. It's so hard to let these things go, God, to offer to others the same grace that I've received when my own words have been harmful to someone else. Help me to remember that while my pregnancy journey hasn't offered much to laugh about, most people don't realize that. God, I pray you would keep me safe from pregnancy narratives that cause me emotional pain. And if people slip up, keep my heart from growing bitter.

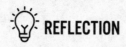 **REFLECTION**

In what ways, if any, are you harboring bitterness toward others who have made careless comments regarding pregnancy? How does understanding your own need for grace and compassion influence the way you feel about that person?

 LETTER

Write a letter to your own heart to share the hurtful things you've heard or seen in relation to pregnancy. How have these words and messages made you feel? How did you respond? In what ways, if any, do you wish you had responded differently? Even now, how might you extend grace and compassion to yourself as well as to those whose words hurt you?

Day 27

THE COURAGE TO CARRY ON IN YOUR WEAKNESS AND GOD'S STRENGTH

But he said to me, "My grace is sufficient for you,
for my power is made perfect in weakness."

—2 Corinthians 12:9

"I don't know how I'm going to get through the day!" I said through sobs as Luke stood in front of the bathroom mirror, preparing to leave for work. With daylight spilling in through the window and what seemed like 10,000-watt light bulbs suspended above me, the room seemed too bright and cheery a spot for my breakdown.

But there I was, falling apart on the edge of the bathtub, with enough tears falling to fill it right to the top.

It was a month before my due date and three weeks before my scheduled induction. Hadn't I come too far for this? Too far to be falling apart when I was *so* close to, hopefully, meeting my baby? It's not as if my emotions had exactly been stable for the past eighteen months, maybe especially for the past eight. I'd hoped that once my due date was within reach, a peace would settle over me, allowing me to power through the remainder of my pregnancy with strength and dignity. But crumbling to pieces in the bathroom on an average Wednesday morning, lips blubbering, limbs flailing, and face hysterical, was far from the image of strength and dignity I'd hoped for.

The look on my husband's face was a combination of concern and empathy as I croaked out a long list of jumbled complaints and irrational fears.

In that moment, along with a million others, I felt beyond weak.

"I'm going to take the day off work," he stated matter-of-factly, without prompting. I was relieved I wouldn't have to face the day alone, and grateful he would be home to care for Annabel and for me. But I hated that so much of his energy was spent tending to me when, as a grown and capable woman, I should have been able to take care of myself. I was tired of needing to be taken care of. And I was tired of being the weak link always on the verge of snapping.

For the third time in my life, my weakness was inescapably obvious. I couldn't hide it, deny it, or manipulate it. It was just *there*—a visibly obvious part of me, no matter how much I wanted it to be different. The first two times involved losing babies and the realization that in my human limitation, I truly wasn't strong enough to control every aspect of my body or the babies formed within it.

As for this time? Well, I was painfully aware that even if I did everything right, I didn't have the power to ensure my baby's well-being, even when he was in what was supposed to be the safety of my womb. My pregnancy was slowly creeping to a close and the outlook was optimistic by all accounts (except for my own), but the exhaustion from months of worry had worn me down and full-on panic was settling in because I didn't think I could possibly keep going for another three weeks. And I wasn't sure my baby boy could either.

I stood to look in the bathroom mirror, my gaze moving from my tearstained face down to my enormous belly, which was bursting with life. Yet, I was on the verge of imploding.

We were so close to the finish line of the longest, slowest race of my life, yet my whole body threatened to buckle under the weight of uncertainty I'd carried for so long. I wanted to run toward that finish line with vigor, hurrying toward the assumption that a thriving baby would be waiting there for me, my prize for sticking it out and reaching the end. Instead, I limped, weary from the heaviness of grief and worry, the only certainty being that I could make no assumptions. Bringing a baby home seemed as unlikely now as it had eight months ago, when the lines of a pregnancy test signaled that the race had begun.

The night before my edge-of-the-tub meltdown, I had been comforted by the sensation of my baby moving. I was amazed that I could actually differentiate between his knees and his fists as he stretched his body and my belly as far as he possibly could. His birth—his life—was so close I could taste it; the sweet drink of hope I needed to keep going.

But by morning, that sense of comfort had faded, leaving my mouth dry and once again in search of sustenance. The reassurance from the night before seemed like a distant memory as a sense of panic flooded the bathroom. For thirty-six weeks, my body had carried a baby boy who was still demonstrating his will to survive, yet the rolling anxiety left me parched instead of sipping on hope from the night before. *Does he have another three weeks in him? Do I?*

I was physically weak and emotionally wrecked, tossed around by waves of the unknown. I wanted to be a beacon of strength, but I was just treading water and tiring quickly, with little energy to keep going. So close, but still impossibly far away. And still without a promise of what lay before me.

I felt foolish hunched over on the edge of that bathtub, crying and scared, when there really wasn't a good reason to be. Everything was fine, wasn't it? Not one of the concerns that had been raised during my pregnancy had resulted in actual complications. But that's part of why pregnancy after loss is so hard. I knew that there didn't have to be any defined or actualized complications for my pregnancy to unravel into a pile of tattered hopes and broken dreams.

I felt utterly deficient, just as I had after losing Micah. Too weak to keep going, to keep hoping that something good awaited on the other side. And while I wish I could say that I glided through my pregnancy gracefully—without the tears and brokenness and debilitating anxiety—the good news is, I didn't have to.

And neither do you.

Because God's grace is more than enough to make up for whatever we lack. It's in our weakness that we see his strength. He lifts us from our edge-of-the-bathtub meltdowns, and as we lean on him when our bodies are tired and unsteady, he's enough when we're not.

Maybe you *are* sailing gracefully through your pregnancy instead of treading water and trying to stay afloat like I was. Maybe you *have* reached your stride as you steadily and confidently power toward the finish line. But it could also be that your pregnancy has been more of a limp than a nimble stride, more of a gasping for air from the waves of anxiety than steady breathing as you glide along. If so, I understand.

I got up from the edge of the tub that morning, not with steady feet or measured breathing, but with a vulnerability that said, *I can't do this alone.*

And that takes courage. To admit our weakness and cry out for relief.

When my husband stepped in, so did God, sustaining me with his grace and provision when I was too weak to face another uncertain day on my own.

We don't have to pick ourselves up out of a pool of tears in our own strength because we were made to rely on God. We are made to focus on his strength instead of our weakness, trusting that he is enough.

> Look to the LORD and his strength. (1 Chronicles 16:11)

Friend, when fear and weakness bring you to your knees, position your weary body against the steady presence of the Lord and rely on his boundless strength. It's in our weakness that his might becomes evident. You don't have to navigate this season perfectly or with the perceived gracefulness of other pregnant women. You are allowed to break down because his grace is sufficient when you can't do this on your own.

And it takes courage to admit that you can't.

God, never have I been more aware of my weaknesses than through this experience of loss and pregnancy after loss. I'm so tired of falling apart due to the stress and fear of the unknown. I thought that as I got closer to my due date, my fears would decrease. Instead, the closer I get, the more I worry. It's still so hard to believe that I might actually bring my baby home. While I'm so grateful for this chapter you've written into my life, I'm also ready for it to be over—I'm ready to move forward with my baby in my arms. I see other women gliding gracefully through their pregnancies while I continue to limp, and I wish this experience were easier for me. So often I wish I could be more like them, but you remind me that I don't have to be because your grace is sufficient, and your strength is enough to pick me up when I fall to my knees. God, I'm getting closer, but I need your strength to keep going.

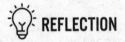 **REFLECTION**

In what ways have you felt weak during your pregnancy? Even now, what would it mean for you to admit your weakness and cry out for help and relief? How do you need God to match your weakness with his strength?

 LETTER

Tell your baby how you have experienced, or how you hope to experience, God's strength and grace as you journey through pregnancy.

Day 28

THE COURAGE TO TRUST THE GOD OF RESTORATION

In his hand is the life of every creature
and the breath of all mankind.

—JOB 12:10

I'm not one to put much stock in perceived signs from above. But I do believe God places small, unexpected tokens of beauty in our path as tangible proof that he is present and that his goodness endures despite unwelcome circumstances. They may not be signs, but they do remind us that he is so much bigger than the valleys we travel through, greater than the intimidating journey we face as we traverse dark paths and blind curves on our way to the destination of healthy-newborn-baby land.

It was April, and I was nearing the dawn of the third trimester. But while my calendar insisted it was spring, the clouds protested by unleashing a blast of snow that carpeted the earth in white. It wasn't the first episode of treacherous weather that spring and it wouldn't be the last. The green grass peeked out from beneath the thinning layers of snow just long enough to tease me with the promise of a life in bloom before retreating back beneath the thick, cold sheet of winter again.

My pregnancy was moving forward, but I remained stranded in the precarious season between winter and summer, loss and life. I was becoming increasingly frustrated by the lack of warmth, sunshine, and color. I needed open windows and fresh air, buds in bloom and fragrant flowers to prove to me that life could emerge from the sleep of death and dirt. Because I wasn't so sure anymore. I was still waiting for new life to spring forth from my body, but like the earth and air in April, I couldn't hurry the process along. The lengthy days of waiting would have to run their course.

Like the world around me, in many ways I actually was starting to come back to life. I had made an appointment for maternity photos. I had purchased a few small baby items. We had decided to move (which, by the way, I do *not* recommend doing during an already beyond-stressful season), and I was cautiously imagining a fresh start in a new house with a new baby. I was starting to make tentative plans, though reluctantly, because like the spring weather, I couldn't say definitively what was in store from one day to the next. I was without a doubt still enduring the season of pregnancy, but I remained in a state of limbo, the signs of life there but simultaneously hidden.

On one particularly snowy spring morning, I stood at the window in a thick sweater, my arms hugging my body in an effort to stave off the cold. Suspended between a white earth and gray sky, I lamented the slow pace at which life was moving. In a season of chilling uncertainty, the possibilities as bleak as they were promising, it wasn't fast enough.

How much longer, Lord? How much longer until the ground thaws? How much longer until color emerges from the blank canvas of winter? How much longer until a warm-bodied baby thaws the bitterness that has paralyzed me for so long? How much longer until the gloom disperses and life feels good again?

And then I saw it. A sliver of green next to a droplet of magenta, a sight that was out of place amid the colorless landscape. It was the tip of a tulip that had pushed its way through winter's suffocating blanket, a tulip I'd seen before but hadn't expected to see again.

More than a year prior, I'd been given a potted tulip after Micah died. It was a small but not insignificant bright spot during those early days of dark grief. My favorite flower, given to me by a friend who didn't know the fondness I held for those delicately curved petals. It was one of those unexpected glimmers of beauty that appeared on the dreadful road of grief, a reminder that even though my friend didn't know that small, personal detail about me, God did, and he revealed himself to me through the gesture of that small gift.

However, after a couple of weeks in bloom, it hadn't taken long for the potted tulip to shrivel. In my own state of grief-induced deterioration, I simply left the bulb on the countertop to die. Over time it became a skeleton, a withered, dried-out shell of the life it once held.

When my parents came to visit months later, my father, a skilled gardener, buried that pitiful bulb deep in the dirt of our front yard.

"I don't know that it will come up next year," he said. "It might be too warm already and the bulb might be too far gone." Like pregnancy, there were no guarantees. I carried on without thinking of it again. My mental energy was focused on only two thoughts: how to survive the loss of Micah and how to pursue the possibility of another baby being planted in my womb.

Now, less than a year later, I gazed at the bright petals of that reborn tulip and remembered my low expectations for that small, crumbling bulb. I was in awe because it had defied its once-withered state as well as the relentless snowfall that had the power to destroy the fragile petals of early spring. Once more, my eyes met a small token of beauty on what had been a dark and burdensome road.

It was almost as if that flower was God's response to my lament; as if God's answer to my *How much longer?* was a tender *Not much.*

I can't say that this was the moment I knew everything was going to work out. To be honest, I never really had that moment. Nor did I assume that the survival of a single plant under less-than-ideal circumstances was a sign that my baby would also survive. But I did consider that if that little tulip could defy the odds, maybe my baby could too.

It wasn't a promise, but I did accept it as a symbol of life, of hope.

This was God, producing life where there had been none. And if he cared enough to resurrect a simple flower, how much more did he care about me? My life? The life of my baby?

During my pregnancy, I had felt joy each time my baby stirred. But as I fixed my eyes on that tiny burst of color, I could see it—joy cropping up from desolation. And I could sense God's goodness as well as his sovereignty.

Maybe in this drawn-out season of hardship, you're in search of something similar. A sign. Maybe you're looking for evidence that God is near and powerful, just as he says he is. Or maybe you want a reason to trust him when he's allowed so much to be taken from you. It certainly isn't easy to trust much of anything when you've lost a baby and the ground you once thought to be sturdy crumbles and crashes down around you.

And the God of all grace, who called you to his eternal glory in Christ, after you have suffered a little while, will himself restore you and make you strong, firm and steadfast. (1 Peter 5:10)

Even so, may I encourage you to look around, friend? Every beautiful life you see is in and of God's hands. He doesn't take your life or the life within you lightly. He is trustworthy even when you haven't rounded the curve that allows you to see what the end of this road holds. His specialty is restoration despite awful and seemingly impossible circumstances. If your surroundings seem lacking in the beauty that you long for during this unpredictable and perhaps harsh season, might you cling to the beauty of that truth?

God, there was a time when I trusted my body. A time when I trusted the process of pregnancy. A time when I easily trusted you. But loss has changed all that. Grief has often overshadowed the beauty around me, and hardship has hampered the joy I once associated with pregnancy. I keep wondering how much longer this hard season is going to last. I want to feel refreshed, restored. Yet, I'm still waiting for the clouds to clear, for the beauty to return without grief and anxiety as my constant companions. I know that you are the God of all living things and that you are trustworthy even when life doesn't go as planned. Help me to see the beauty in this truth and to trust that the loss I've experienced will one day be restored. Open my eyes to the joy in the small graces and gifts you provide. I can't see what's around the curve, but help me to believe that you are already there and greater than whatever may lie ahead of me.

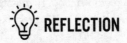

REFLECTION

In what ways have you noticed or felt God's presence during this season? What tokens of beauty has God placed in your path?

LETTER

Describe for your baby the beauty that you can see today—right now—whether or not it's pregnancy related.

Day 29

THE COURAGE TO (FINALLY) SURRENDER

LORD, *I know that people's lives are not their
own;
it is not for them to direct their steps.*
—JEREMIAH 10:23

I'd known for a long time what little control I possessed, yet
a part of me continued to believe I had the ability to mold my
pregnancy into a masterpiece, one in which the final presentation
would be a glowing representation of life rather than a stark and
somber depiction of death. *If I just do this, this, and that, maybe I can
shape my pregnancy into a fully formed, pink-skinned baby who can be
seen, touched, and physically present in our home.*

But deep down, I knew the fate of the masterpiece forming
inside me wasn't truly in my hands. In fact, before becoming pregnant again, I surrendered my circumstances to God—though not
until I'd grieved to the point of sorrow dripping from every pore
at the realization that I couldn't outrun loss and grief or predict

the future. I had grown so tired of obsessing over the questions of *why* and *when*.

Why me, God? Why did I have to lose my baby? Why not her? Why have two of my pregnancies failed? Why was I chosen to give birth to a baby who was already dead? Why did you allow Micah to be taken away from me? When, God? When will it be my turn to bring another life into the world? When will I get to hold another baby? When will the tears dry up and the grief end?

I felt entrenched in a pit of muck that was churning with unknowns and unanswered questions, grief, and groaning. I'd been obsessed with finding a way out and I was so, so tired of fighting, of trying to make sense out of circumstances that made no sense, of wondering when life would take a turn for the better. Which led me to the solitude of a steam room one day, uttering a message of surrender to God.

"I can't do this anymore!" I cried. "I surrender! I surrender it all to you. This whole situation. My longing for another baby. My attempts to control the timing of adding to our family, or anything at all. I surrender!"

I finally felt like I could breathe. I felt a peace I hadn't felt in a long time. At least, I did until I became pregnant again. That's when thoughts of blood and death and emptiness practically jumped off the tiny window of the positive pregnancy test, birthing an anxiety so consuming I felt desperate to contain it. My attempts to keep my imagined fears from becoming actual events were immediately thrust into action, though I knew that's all they were. Attempts. Not assurances.

Even so, my feelings told me it was entirely up to me to see my pregnancy through to a live birth. Efforts to control the outcome were my coping mechanism. I requested early and extra appointments. I stayed off my feet. I hired help to care for Annabel. I left most of the household duties to Luke. I enlisted the help of family and friends to take over daily tasks, chores, and errands. I put off sex based on my history of loss and fear that it might in some way interfere with my pregnancy. I tried so hard to do everything right, which seemed to be paying off as my pregnancy steadily, though not effortlessly, progressed through the third trimester.

When my midwife offered me the option to induce labor a week before my due date, I gladly took it, considering it an answered prayer. It's safe to say I was relieved, but it wasn't without a trace of smugness. There was a part of me that felt I was being compensated for the hard work of trying to control every aspect of my pregnancy.

I had a date. The official countdown had begun, and I could mark the calendar for my baby's arrival. I was just six weeks away from meeting my son.

Except, when the time came, things didn't go as planned.

Despite being in the hospital for two days, my body pumped full of synthetic oxytocin and other labor-inducing medications, my body refused to go into labor. Apparently, no amount of human-made medicine could make my stubborn cervix budge. Had I not begun crying at the midwife's news that I was being released, I would have laughed at the irony of it all. For months, we'd closely monitored my cervix out of concern that it might give out early, too early for my baby's life to even be considered viable. And now here I was, my pregnancy having reached full term, and we couldn't force it open with an excess of powerful drugs that were made for that very thing.

From the moment I found out I was pregnant, I assumed

nothing. Until, at eight days shy of my due date, I checked into the hospital fully believing that, if nothing else, I'd walk out of there a day or two later having given birth. Because labor induction was a sure thing, right? After all, I'd been induced with my first pregnancy, and while it was a slow, arduous process, it culminated in our family of two increasing to three. It was the one guarantee I had. Or so I thought.

For forty-some hours as I awaited the birth of my son, medical staff hustled about the labor and delivery unit, stopping in my room to check on my progress (or lack thereof), repeatedly informing me that the floor was busier than usual. The midwives tending to me were so often interrupted to assist with other deliveries that I lost track of how many babies were born during my stay. The floor was a symphony of high-pitched wails and suckling mouths, signaling the inauguration of numerous women who were stepping into the role of mothering their new child.

I'm going to be next, I thought, each time I heard that another baby was born. But my place in line was further back than I realized.

"I know you're anxious to have this baby," the midwife said, "but labor hasn't progressed at all. That happens sometimes, and there's nothing we can do about it."

It wasn't just that labor hadn't progressed—it hadn't even *started*. She assured me that my baby boy was healthy, noting his steady heart rate and patterns of movement. "He's just not ready to come out yet," she said. "So we're going to discharge you, and who knows? Maybe you'll go into labor on your own tomorrow!"

That note of cheery optimism was nauseating, though I know it was meant to encourage me. I wanted to shake her and beg her to get my baby out of me before something happened to him. I would have gleefully agreed to a C-section, even though I knew it wasn't warranted. There was no emergency, just a scared mama stuck in the crises of her past.

Tears welled up in my eyes and before turning to leave, the midwife squeezed my hand and whispered, "I'm sorry," as I silently pleaded for her to change her mind and invite me to stay.

With that, Luke and I shuffled out to the car, no closer to holding our son than when we'd arrived, and it was disheartening to say the least. I hoisted my unbalanced body into the passenger's seat, and instead of marveling at how small my baby was in the infant car seat we'd installed in the back of the car, I examined my enlarged belly and wondered how much longer he could survive in there.

We'd been confident that a scheduled induction, a relatively common approach to the birth process, was within our control, having faith that it was the answer to a long and strenuous pregnancy. But perhaps our faith had been misplaced when the failed induction proved once again that God was the only one in control.

As we drove home, I found myself sinking into that familiar pit of muck, only this time surrounded by different questions involving a different scenario. Again, I assumed a posture of surrender.

Fine, God. Fine. There's nothing else I can do, anyway. He'll be born when he's supposed to be born. I trust you. I'm giving it all to you because I'm tired of thinking about it.

And it was true. Mostly. I *wanted* it to be true, at least. If nothing else, I trusted that my desire to *want* to trust God's plan and timing counted for something.

I had done everything right, and just when I was about to collect what I figured I'd earned, the payoff got pushed back. The timing was off. The plan changed. And I felt deceived.

Maybe you feel that way too. Like you've done the right things, made good choices, done your best to trust God, only to be let down. Maybe things still aren't going your way even though you've tried so hard to steer your pregnancy in that direction.

If so, remember this: we have a God who knows us better than we know ourselves. He knows where we're going even when we don't, which is why we can be comforted even when our sense of control dissolves in our hands. There is comfort when we realize that our pregnancies are in hands far steadier than our own, and that our lives are being formed into something good even when we feel defeated.

> He knows us far better than we know ourselves, knows our
> pregnant condition, and keeps us present before God. That's
> why we can be so sure that every detail in our lives of love for
> God is worked into something good. (Romans 8:27–28 MSG)

It's not easy to accept because we are so deeply invested in the process of bringing life into the world. As mothers, *of course we are.* We were made to invest our energy in the children we mother, whether or not they've been born. But without investing our hope and trust in God, without surrendering to his plans and timing, we won't have the comfort and reassurance we need. Our attempts to control what can't be controlled are never enough to bring us the peace we desire.

Maybe like me you've relinquished control only to pick it back up again. But I've come to realize that the act of surrender isn't a one-and-done decision. It's a daily process. Because we have a hard time keeping our hands off the reins, don't we? But our hands aren't actually the ones operating them.

And knowing that, we can let go and surrender our plans to God, knowing he is working for our good even when our plans fail.

God, surrender sometimes sounds like a foreign word to me. I want to be in control and like to think that I am—at least some of the time. But my failed plans have proven that's not the case. I get stuck thinking I know what's best and that it's completely up to me to determine my baby's future, which is interesting because that hasn't worked for me in the past. Through Scripture and circumstances, you remind me that it's you who is in control, whose plans never fail—and never fail to be good. God, I don't want to loosen my grip on the reins of my pregnancy—because it's my pregnancy, isn't it? But the truth is, this baby first belonged to you. Help me to surrender my child to you, because you know me better than I know myself.

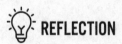 **REFLECTION**

In what ways have your attempts to control things during this or a previous pregnancy failed to serve you? What can you surrender to God today?

 LETTER

Describe for your baby the ways you've seen God work in his or her favor since you became pregnant.

Day 30

COURAGEOUSLY BELIEVING THAT JOY WILL COME IN THE MORNING—EVEN IF

Weeping may tarry for the night,
but joy comes with the morning.

—PSALM 30:5 ESV

Maybe you've sensed it while reading through the previous chapters. My baby boy, the product of my fourth pregnancy, did in fact come home with me. He is the sibling my daughter can play with and the second baby to whom Luke and I didn't have to say goodbye.

Two weeks after my failed induction, I returned to the hospital to be induced for a second time. It was a week past my due date, and even after having my membranes stripped multiple times, drinking cup after cup of raspberry leaf tea, taking long walks, and gorging on as much spicy food as I could handle, labor evaded me.

The physical baggage I walked into the hospital with was

205

lighter than what I'd carried when giving birth to Annabel, but the emotional baggage was far heavier. I wasn't aiming for a natural birth as I had been before. I didn't have the desire to bring a selection of clothing to choose from for both my own and my baby's going-home outfits—you know, depending on the weather and my mood. I no longer lived under the illusion that having a plan would make for a desirable birth experience. The only thing I cared about was bringing my baby safely into the world, and if it took medication or even surgery to do so, that was fine by me. Which is why I left behind the essential oils, handheld massager, excess clothing, and birth plan.

Instead, I walked through the sliding-glass hospital doors carrying the weight of two losses, memories of ultrasounds that showed no life, and hospital rooms that remained silent after a baby was born. For the two and a half years after loss first entered my life, I'd been lugging around grief and uncertainty and endless questions about what would come next. And I'd been waiting for a chance to again enter the hospital in expectation of new life rather than confirmation of death.

Fifteen hours after I arrived, the wait was over.

At 12:08 a.m., on July 28, 2016, my son Aksel was born. And while I'm sure he released a deafening shriek, I don't remember it. All I know is that upon his arrival, I immediately asked my midwife if he was okay, and she responded by placing his warm body against mine. The sound of his breathing was my answer.

Now, I'm guessing that this may be one in a series of success stories you've read or heard as you wait on your own successful birth story, your own breathing baby. Just as I did so many times, you might be thinking, *That's great for her, but I might not be so lucky.*

But these stories? These babies you see and hear about? They are proof of possibility. They are demonstrations of hope. They show us that joy does come in the morning, though it's true that it might not look the same for all of us.

I could rattle off some statistics to encourage you that the odds of having a healthy baby are in your favor. But I won't. Because, like you, I know better than to assume that good odds equal happy endings. Even after multiple losses, not everyone gets the ending they want.

Shortly after Aksel was born, an acquaintance who was pregnant after having a miscarriage reached full term only to give birth to a stillborn baby girl. She'd carried two babies and lost them both. It was heartbreaking, unfair, and confusing. As I rocked my living baby, I looked at photos she'd shared online of her stillborn child and mourned with her from a distance, wishing I could take away her pain. My prayers had been answered, and I desperately wanted to know why hers had not.

Once again I was reminded that loss doesn't discriminate. It doesn't care if you've already endured more than your share of heartache. It can come for you at any time.

I don't say these things to bring you down. I say them simply to acknowledge that I wrote this book with an awareness that not everyone will experience the same ending as mine. At least, not in their own timing. I don't want to ignore that reality because it's a hard truth many women will face.

Each of our stories is going to read differently. Some of us have only had pregnancies that ended in loss. Some of us gave birth to healthy children before the chapters of loss were written. Some of us go on to have multiple successful pregnancies. Some of us decide to stop trying before we really feel ready to. And some of us continue taking steps toward the possibility of another baby for longer than we thought we could, despite crippling fear, hoping that there's still space on the page to write the ending we want.

I've often wondered where I would be in my journey of loss and life after if Aksel hadn't made it home. Would we have tried again? Would we have accepted our status as parents to one living child? Would we have explored adoption? I don't know.

But I do know this: even if Aksel hadn't made it home, joy would still be on the horizon. And I don't say that lightly. There surely would have been another long season of deep grief. The sorrow would have felt unbearable; the weeping would have nearly drowned me in tears. Very simply, I would've deeply *hated* having to endure another loss. But the joy of morning—after mourning—would still have come, even if not in the way I envisioned it.

> Those who sow with tears
> will reap with songs of joy. (Psalm 126:5)

Even if my son had entered heaven instead of earth, I would still have found joy in being his mother, even if not right away. Like his siblings who passed through the pearly gates, he would have left a beautiful mark on my life, and I would have found ways to make his short life meaningful. I know this because I felt the same way with the babies I lost.

And further down the road, the big, life-changing joy would come with our reunion in the glory of heaven, just as it will with the two who are there now. Even if my son had died, I would still have the hope of heaven and the promise of no more bone-crushing grief.

He will wipe every tear from their eyes. There will be no more death or mourning or crying or pain, for the old order of things has passed away. (Revelation 21:4)

Sweet friend, I cannot predict how this chapter of your story will end, but I am praying wholeheartedly that it wraps up with you joyfully leaving the hospital with your baby. I hope the success stories of the ones who have gone before you are a source of hope rather than cause for envy or despair. I'm praying that your morning comes sooner rather than later and that it looks and sounds like the wail of a healthy newborn baby.

But even if your prayers for this baby aren't answered in the way you desire, this pregnancy will have been worth it. Because your baby's life matters, as does your love for your precious little one. Even if you find yourself carrying the grief of another loss, we know that it's temporary—miserable, unwelcome, and devastating, but temporary.

Because the things of this world, including the pain, aren't going to last forever. God promises to restore every broken thing, including your motherhood. And I hope that no matter what happens, you can find the courage to believe that.

God, oh, how I look forward to the arrival of morning! I'm praying that it involves the radiance of new life looking up at me from the embrace of my arms. I hear so many stories of healthy babies being born after loss, and it gives me hope that the same is possible for me. However, I still fear the worst because I know we don't always get the ending we want on earth. I thank you for this baby, no matter what, God. And I thank you for the promise that pure joy is on the horizon—that one day all the heartache of this earth will vanish—for one day I will hold all of my babies in heaven. I trust you to restore my motherhood, and I trust you to hold my baby close, whether in heaven or on earth.

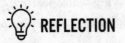

REFLECTION

How do you respond to the idea that joy is on the horizon, no matter what the outcome of your pregnancy might be?

LETTER

Tell your baby all the ways you will love him or her and how this pregnancy has impacted you for the better—even if.

ACKNOWLEDGMENTS

If there's one thing I've learned, it's that God keeps his promises. He has used some of the very worst times in my life for more good than I could have imagined. Time and again, he's shown me that he is here and that he is working, even in the heartbreak and indescribable mess. After I lost Micah, God whispered that he was going to do something with my story, but I didn't really believe it, nor could I imagine what that could possibly mean. Now I do. This book is my story, but made possible only by him. God, thank you for your endless love and grace.

Luke, thank you for always putting me first. You love me sacrificially every single day. We have walked some dark roads together, but by God's grace have always come back into the light. This book wouldn't have been possible without your love, support, and patience. There's no one I'd rather do life with than you. I love you.

Annabel and Aksel. My sunshine and my rainbow. Thank you for giving me grace always. Most days I still can't believe that God made you mine. I love you both.

To my parents: Thank you for being there when life was falling apart. Your excitement about this book brings me joy (though

ACKNOWLEDGMENTS

I still can't help but roll my eyes when you talk about it—sorry,
Mom).

To my in-laws: Thank you for raising your son into a good
man, whom I now get to call mine. Your support has not gone
unnoticed.

Thanks to my agent, Blythe Daniel, for believing in this message and for taking a chance on me. Working with you has been
nothing short of wonderful. Your expertise has been invaluable,
and your encouragement a gift.

Thank you, Jessica Wong Rogers, for immediately seeing my
vision for this book and for understanding the need for it. While
we weren't able to work together for long, thank you for making
Nelson Books home. Jenny Baumgartner, thank you for jumping
right in on this project. Your kindness and humor are treasures and
you've helped make this book better. Lauren Langston Stewart
and the entire team at Nelson Books, thank you for your hard
work and dedication in bringing this book to life.

To the Pregnancy After Loss Support team: Thank you for
sharing the hard stories that need to be told. Lindsey Henke, thank
you for creating a safe and supportive place for mamas who have
experienced the worst kind of loss, a place where grief meets hope.
Valerie Meek, thank you for publishing my words for the very first
time (and many times since then). I'll never forget seeing your
name in my in-box that day; you were a virtual stranger who has
become a real friend.

To the entire Her View from Home team: This book wouldn't
have been possible without your ongoing support and encouragement. Thank you for always teaching me and for helping me grow.
Leslie Means, thank you for passionately sharing our stories with
the world. You are an exemplary leader. Carolyn Moore, thank

you for publishing my words for the second time (and many times after). I'm forever grateful for the invitation into this community. Whitney Fleming, thank you for tirelessly pouring into the women on this team and for helping nurture this book idea. I've no doubt that you are the result of God's plan and timing. And to all those at Homestock who encouraged me to leap into the book-writing process, thank you.

To the friends who listened to me hesitantly talk about this book when it was nothing more than an idea: Thank you for your enthusiasm and for believing in it from the start. But mostly, thank you for not laughing. You never doubted me, and that means everything.

Mikala, thank you for faithfully walking with me on this wild journey of publishing an actual book. You've never failed to listen and have made this all so much fun. I'm so grateful for your friendship.

Jenn, thank you for your early guidance and feedback on the words and Scripture included in this book. Your wisdom is a gift.

Lisa, thank you for every single text, phone call, and pep talk. You emanate nothing but love and kindness.

Brynn, thank you for the endless laughs and the early input on what has now become a book.

To my readers: Thank you for reading my words. Your support and encouragement have made this book possible. You are so darn kind, and I'm humbled that you keep showing up. I'm grateful to be the keeper of so many of your stories.

To every mama who has experienced loss: I am so sorry. I wish there were never a need for a book like this. Not one of us ever wanted to say goodbye to a precious baby. Not one of us ever wanted to spend a subsequent pregnancy in fear of saying goodbye to another. I admire your courage, of which it takes much, to keep going. I'm confident that God isn't done with you yet. Thank you for sharing your stories and for showing up for mine.

NOTES

1. Brené Brown, *Daring Greatly: How the Courage to Be Vulnerable Transforms the Way We Live, Love, Parent, and Lead* (New York: Gotham Books, 2012), 126.
2. "Pregnancy After Miscarriage," American Pregnancy Association, April 25, 2012, https://americanpregnancy.org/getting-pregnant/pregnancy-loss/pregnancy-after-miscarriage-71034/.

ABOUT THE AUTHOR

Jenny Albers is a wife, mother, and writer. She is the founder of Still Loved, an online community that exists to amplify the voices of parents who have experienced the loss of a pregnancy or infant. Her writing, which focuses on pregnancy loss, motherhood, and faith, has been featured at Pregnancy After Loss Support, Her View from Home, Today Parents, and a variety of other online publications. She lives in South Dakota with her husband and two living children.

You can connect with Jenny at www.JennyAlbers.com or by searching @jennyalbersauthor on social media.